RESEARCH ETHICS
IN THE REAL WORLD:
ISSUES AND SOLUTIONS FOR
HEALTH AND SOCIAL CARE

T0249661

For Elsevier:

Publisher: Steven Black
Development Editors: Dinah Thom and Gillian Cloke
Project Manager: Nancy Arnott
Design Direction: George Ajayi

RESEARCH ETHICS
IN THE REAL WORLD:
Issues and solutions for health and social care

Tony Long BSc (Hons) MA PhD RN

Professor of Child and Family Health, University of Salford Centre for Nursing, Midwifery and Collaborative Research, Salford, UK

Martin Johnson MSc PhD RN

Professor in Nursing and Director of the University of Salford Centre for Nursing, Midwifery and Collaborative Research, Salford, UK

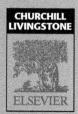

CHURCHILL
LIVINGSTONE

ELSEVIER

Edinburgh   London   New York   Oxford   Philadelphia   St Louis   Sydney   Toronto   2007

CHURCHILL LIVINGSTONE
ELSEVIER

First published 2007

ISBN 10: 0-44-3-10065-9
ISBN 13: 978-0-443-10065-9

British Library Cataloguing in Publication Data
A catalogue record for this book is available from the British Library

Library of Congress Cataloging in Publication Data
A catalog record for this book is available from the Library of Congress

Notice
Medical knowledge is constantly changing. Standard safety precautions must be followed, but as new research and clinical experience broaden our knowledge, changes in treatment and drug therapy may become necessary or appropriate. Readers are advised to check the most current product information provided by the manufacturer of each drug to be administered to verify the recommended dose, the method and duration of administration, and contraindications. It is the responsibility of the practitioner, relying on experience and knowledge of the patient, to determine dosages and the best treatment for each individual patient. Neither the Publisher nor the editors nor contributors assume any liability for any injury and/or damage to persons or property arising from this publication.

The Publisher

Transferred to digital printing in 2009.

Contents

Contributors

Debbie Fallon RN, RSCN, MA is Senior Lecturer within the child health team in the University of Salford School of Nursing and Salford Centre for Nursing, Midwifery and Collaborative Research. Her research interests have focused particularly on adolescent experiences of sexual health services in a sociological context. She is currently completing a PhD entitled *Accessing emergency contraception – a feminist analysis of the adolescent experience* at Goldmith's College, London.

Carol Haigh RN, MSc, PhD is Senior Lecturer in Research for The University of Salford Centre for Nursing, Midwifery and Collaborative Research in Greater Manchester. Her research interests include pain management and chaos theory. She has published widely on the topic of techno-research and cyber ethics.

Michelle Howarth RN, MSc, PGCE (Dist) is Lecturer in Nursing at the University of Salford where she is involved in the *Shaping the Future* Project funded by the Northwest Development Agency. She has a clinical practitioner background in medical nursing, which she practised for 9 years. She also worked as a Research & Development Co-ordinator at Bury Acute NHS Trust. Her research interests include integrated health and social care and gerontology.

Martin Johnson RN, MSc, PhD is Professor in Nursing and Director of The University of Salford Centre for Nursing, Midwifery and Collaborative Research in Greater Manchester. His *Nursing Power and Social Judgement*, Ashgate, Aldershot (1997) examined the social context of a hospital ward, offering insights into the way that nurses and their patients negotiate, or struggle, for the power to achieve their goals through judgemental labelling. He has published widely on research ethics and recently chaired a group producing the Royal College of Nursing's new Guidance on Research Ethics in Nursing.

Neil Jones RN, MSc, BA (Hons), Cert Ed is Senior Lecturer in the Foundation Studies Division of the Nursing Department at the University of Central Lancashire. Over the past decade the main focus of Neil's work has been with open and distance-learning programmes, particularly E.N. Conversion and degree pathways. He has a keen interest in spirituality and is module leader for the post-registration degree modules 'Spirituality and Health' and 'Environment as a Health Issue'.

Rosie Kneafsey RN, MRes, BSc (Hons) is Lecturer in Nursing at the University of Salford. After completing a degree in nursing at the University of Edinburgh, Rosie worked as a staff nurse in a neurosurgical setting and then a high-dependency unit for head-injured patients. More recently, she worked as a research fellow working on an ENB funded project in the area of rehabilitation. She has a special interest in back injury and its prevention and has published widely on rehabilitation, back injury and research governance issues.

Tony Long RN, BSc (Hons), MA, PhD is Professor of Child and Family Health in the University of Salford Centre for Nursing, Midwifery and Collaborative Research, and Associate Head of School for Research in the School of Nursing. He leads on research with children and families and has published widely in this field, as well as on health professional education and professional regulation. He was co-editor of the recently revised Royal College of Nursing *Research Ethics: Guidance for Nurses*. His book *Excessive Crying in Infancy* offered insights from research into the causes, effects and experiences of families coping with babies who cry persistently.

Tracey Williamson RN, BSc (Hons), MSc PhD is a Research Fellow at the University of Salford. Until 2004 she was a nurse consultant at Pennine Acute Hospitals NHS Trust holding an honorary research fellow position in the Institute for Health and Social Care Research. Her research interests include shared governance, user involvement in research and the care of older people.

Foreword

Ethics in healthcare practice and research is a hot topic. At the time of writing, the BBC is broadcasting the second series of its 'Inside the Ethics Committee' programmes. Each programme focuses on a particular clinical ethical dilemma, and service users, clinicians and ethicists discuss case studies in order to present all sides of the dilemma and give reasons for the outcome.

Turning to ethics in research, a worldwide Google search on 'ethics and the pharmaceutical industry' yields over 10 million sites while, perhaps surprisingly, 'ethics and nursing research' produces over 18 million. Readers of John le Carré's book 'The Constant Gardener', and those who have seen the film version, will readily understand why 'big pharma' features so heavily. Things in this field do not seem to have changed that much since I studied the Report of the Committee of Enquiry into the Relationship of the Pharmaceutical Industry with the National Health Service 1965-1967 (Chairman: Lord Sainsbury) on the drug industry as a sociology undergraduate over 30 years ago.

Perhaps even more tellingly in the light of the content of this book, a worldwide – not just UK – Google search on 'research ethics committee' lists the UK Central Office for Research Ethics Committees (COREC) site (http://www.corec.org.uk/) as number one and Governance Arrangements for NHS Research Ethics Committees as number three. The former is the site where researchers enter the application process and the latter 'provides a standards framework for the process of review of the ethics of all proposals for research in the NHS and Social Care which is efficient, effective and timely, and which will command public confidence. It sets out general standards and principles for an accountable system of Research Ethics Committees, working collaboratively to common high standards of review and operating process throughout the NHS (http://www.dh.gov.uk/PublicationsAndStatistics/Publications/PublicationsPolicyAndGuidance/PublicationsPolicyAndGuidanceArticle/fs/en?CONTENT_ID=4005727&chk=CNcpyR).

Unless people all round the world are accessing these sites to tap into examples of good practice, we must presume that researchers in the UK are using these sites heavily. Since each instance of accessing the sites will be measured as a new hit, it may be that a much smaller number of people are repeatedly accessing the sites in an attempt to get their research ethics applications correct before submitting them. This interpretation would chime with the general position in Long and Johnson's book – that the process is over-bureaucratised and time-consuming. If NHS staff wish to complete questionnaires for healthcare researchers in their own time, why is this the business of their employers? Is it not patronising to suggest that these professionals cannot make their own decisions about research participation?

My experience of approaching Local Research Ethics Committees (LRECs) and Multi-Centre Research Ethics (MRECs) is broadly similar to what the contributors to this book suggest – although they sometimes express this in their characteristically forthright style! Nevertheless, I am not sure that their proposed solution – greater reliance on peer review to guarantee ethical research conduct – would solve all the problems. And to be fair, neither do they. However, I am more cynical than they are about ethical behaviour and codes of practice in the social sciences. For example, in one UK university I have come across the situation where undergraduate psychology students are denied access to departmental research resources for their dissertations if they do not participate as subjects in staff research projects – Stanley Milgram would be proud of them!

The contributors to *Research Ethics in the Real World* have addressed these and many other 'real world' ethical issues in a down-to-earth approach that may not be popular with more traditional thinkers. They do not claim to provide definitive answers to the many ethical dilemmas they pose, for debates about research ethics will continue as long as healthcare technology and research approaches themselves continue developing, as illustrated by the chapter by Haigh and Jones on 'Techno-research and cyber ethics: research using the Internet'. Nevertheless the book is a step forward from the more traditional books on the topic which it is intended to replace.

Christine Webb PhD, RN, FRCN
Professor of Health Studies, University of Plymouth, UK
Executive Editor, *Journal of Advanced Nursing*
Editor, *Nurse Author & Editor*

Preface

We have known for years that the literature in this field is insufficient and, especially, that there is a need for a range of resources in one convenient place. The editors and contributors each have direct experience of the aspects of research ethics and research management that they analyse. We are working at the boundaries of 'ethics' and many philosophers would smile at the pedantic and minor concerns of much of the ethics bureaucracy we are at pains to explain. In the health and social services they see thousands harmed by mistakes and hospital infections, doctors and nurses murdering patients and children known to be at risk coming to very serious harm and death. The public must wonder about our priorities. Nevertheless, the protection of research participants (and themselves) has become a major focus of health- and social-care organizations, which has the useful effect of making us all think more about our reasons for, and methods of, investigation.

Having written articles and editorials from time to time on relevant matters, in 2004 we were invited by the Royal College of Nursing Research Society to update its highly successful research ethics guidance publication for members. We were delighted to write a completely new text and then consult in depth with members and an external panel of experts. Whilst we hope the guide is useful, its word limit merely frustrated us that we were skirting round matters of great complexity. Whilst we largely avoided a 'rules' approach, the guide is but one stepping stone. We thought this book might add a few more. In this respect we are grateful to the Society for its support and interest in research ethics and look forward to their feedback.

Our second major motivation in writing and editing the book arose from exasperation that virtually all we read is in terms of absolutes. We mean statements like 'you must have informed consent', 'everyone must be anonymous', 'all the data must be destroyed' and the notorious Latin phrase 'primum non nocere' (first do no harm). Plausible enough at first sight, texts, codes of conduct and advice to researchers are almost universally framed in this sort of language of principles and rules. Our book proposes, in nearly all of its chapters, a radical but much more realistic consequentialist alternative. We call it 'real-world ethics' because this captures the approach with which almost all actual health- and social-care decisions, practice-based or research, are made. Our aim is to improve the degree to which these decisions are based on a full appreciation of the potential outcomes rather than a '10 commandments' approach.

The book is intended for use by students, practitioners and academics (and all the permutations of these roles that the complexities of modern professional life bring). To do justice to the context of any of the serious issues considered here, it has been necessary to focus largely upon bureaucracy and regulations that will be more familiar to readers from Western Europe, Australia and New Zealand. Nevertheless, the core issues in question will remain of direct relevance to others in the USA, Canada and beyond.

Whilst it is now over a decade since the editors coincidentally joined John Harris's 'value of life' lectures at the University of Manchester, we both acknowledge something of a debt to his challenging thinking on matters of real concern in health care. Whilst we would never succeed in imitating the clarity, power and even humour of his approach, we learned much from it. References appear only where really necessary and we own and take responsibility for the opinions we express. Unlike most other work, we do not shrink from analysing real or published examples in the hope that others will do likewise. We fear that the nursing, social work and allied health professions have some way to go to match the vigorous but impersonal criticism of previous work. Whilst we are far from perfecting the skill we offer examples throughout.

We are particularly indebted in different ways to a number of key influences. Christine Webb and Anne Williams, in different ways, opened our eyes both academically and stylistically to rigour and integrity in writing. Whilst we may yet deal insufficiently with relational or feminist thinking in research ethics, we hopefully open the door to what may eventually materialise as the most 'real-world' approach of all.

As editors we are especially grateful to our co-authors from the University of Salford Centre for Nursing, Midwifery and Collaborative Research who met impossibly short deadlines with incredibly good work. We recognised quickly that we were fortunate indeed to have six colleagues with superior knowledge, previous research and publications in their chapter areas. Each of the contributors and their families made sacrifices to produce the text and for this we are especially grateful. At Elsevier Churchill Livingstone, thanks are due to Dinah Thom who remained patient when things got in the way, Gill Cloke and Steven Black for their encouragement and confidence in the material.

We hope and expect that readers will feed back to us their views, either personally or in the relevant media. We will not please everyone. First, our approach will not suit those looking for a code or rule book. Second, we, too, are learning as we go along. Views we express today will change in time through debate and experience, although our generally consequentialist perspective has been quite resilient, and we think it has both logic and the real world of research on its side. Third, we look forward to empirical work that examines research ethics in more depth; to moving away from the armchair and getting into people's homes, schools, clinics, wards and departments, perhaps even into the ethics committees.

Martin Johnson and Tony Long
Editors

Introduction
Tony Long

With so many research books on the market, why should anyone want to produce yet another? Well, even a brief overview of the existing stock is sufficient to illustrate that the predominant approach is firmly principles-based, citing immutable rules of conduct and avoiding discussion of difficult alternative perspectives. This book is different. It is not a textbook of how to undertake research with a chapter on each step of the standard research process, nor is it a reworking of long-established and rarely questioned ethical tomes in which each problem has a clear and unvarying solution.

Employing an overall consequentialist approach, it offers a collection of different perspectives and insights into the problems faced by researchers both experienced and novice in the real world of ambiguity, uncertainty and multiple options. A risk–benefit analysis view is taken of many issues, allowing that differing solutions will be the most acceptable in a variety of circumstances. Many pearls of wisdom are challenged and alternative viewpoints are proposed. Avoiding the unnecessary use of Latin and obscure philosophical abstraction, the text is presented in plain English, amply illustrated with practical examples and supported by many references to further resources.

In an age when the proposed use of a local questionnaire on staff competence must be scrutinised by a research ethics committee before the study can begin, many of us have come to wonder whether some matters in the management and control of research are so far from the horrors of Nuremburg as to have become wildly disproportionate to the potential harm that might be associated with the study. Few, however, dare openly to question current arrangements. This can lead to polarised views and unthinking responses to ethical issues, itself a state of affairs that is more likely to lead to unethical conduct and failure to protect research participants from harm.

The contributors to this book argue many points that, at first sight and out of context, may seem rather questionable or surprising. For example:

- Consent from participants isn't always necessary for the ethical conduct of research.
- Active efforts should be made to inconvenience disadvantaged groups through facilitating their participation in research.
- Paying individuals to participate in research may be acceptable.
- Respect for autonomy, beneficence, non-maleficence and justice together as the basis for decision-making in research ethics are both insufficient and contradictory, having no place in a book such as this.
- The formula for information sheets provided by COREC (the Central Office for Research Ethics Committees) can be an oppressive instrument.
- More research needs to be undertaken using patients in persistent vegetative state as subjects.
- Consent forms are probably almost useless in research studies.
- Personal relationships between a researcher and a research subject during a study are not always obviously wrong.
- It is imperative that research governance is promoted at all levels.
- Providing too much information to a research ethics committee can be hazardous to a successful application.
- A paternalistic approach may be justified in some covert participatory research.

All of these are debated in the text. Difficult issues are confronted and non-standard responses are often expressed.

The authors, all associated with the University of Salford Centre for Nursing, Midwifery and Collaborative Research, adopt a variety of styles to address their chosen topic. At times, for example, those whose participation is sought in research are referred to as 'service users', at other times as 'research participants', and at yet other times simply as 'the public'. This reflects the complex nature of research in the real world, in which most people's lives are characterised by a variety of roles and in which they become, in turn, vulnerable, empowered, disadvantaged and unique. Certainly, when considering subjects and participants in applied research, one size never fits all. The contents of this book are intended to arm the reader with additional insights, new points of view and stimuli for reflection in order to respond positively and effectively to the equally varied challenges of research in health and social care. Practical strategies are suggested, together with guidance on how to tailor a situation-specific solution for the circumstances that prevail in a context-rich real-world research scenario. In this we offer in equal parts food for thought and practical support.

Chapter 2 is Tracey Williamson's examination of the individual in research, in which she utilises a rights-based approach to evaluate critically notions of user participation in research in a number of roles. The complexity of this apparently simple issue is expounded in a thorough analysis of the varied and sometimes conflicting rights of individuals and groups. She raises important questions such as whether it is ever right to use data when, through repeated consenting procedures, respondents 'withdraw' data. Whilst this position has appeal and might develop trust, an absolute right of any respondent to withdraw consent (and therefore the data collected from them) retrospectively could be quite impractical and have profound implications for many studies. One could take the view that data, once freely and consensually given, are no longer the property of the individual, but that of the researcher. Research integrity could be as much about reporting the facts as saying (or not saying) what those studied might like.

In the third chapter Martin Johnson uses real studies from history and more recent times to work through analyses of three major approaches to research design and execution, demonstrating that research is rarely tidy and neatly contained. Instead, it takes place in a complex amalgam of political, social and professional factors, each in itself a microcosm of ever-varying factors and issues for the researcher to appreciate and manage. He discusses professional socialisation and the extent to which the Foucauldian concept of the 'gaze' illustrates a grave paradox in the researcher–respondent relationship. Whilst many research approaches claim to empower service users, the very act of data collection is part of the web of surveillance through which professionals develop and maintain their power over their clients. The extent to which integrity and altruism can overcome such forces is wholly questionable, yet at least some awareness of these, and the genuine rather than patronising involvement of those studied in research design and the research itself, may begin to equalise things.

I then take up the brief in Chapters 4 and 5 to review the ethical issues faced by researchers, shunning the pseudo-philosophical language to be found elsewhere (non-maleficence, beneficence, primum non-nocere, etc.) and focusing instead on the risks or potential harms to participants. I offer practical guidance as to how to address these issues successfully and in an ethically acceptable manner. Instead of assuming that there are fundamental principles to be preserved at all costs, such as confidentiality, anonymity and, especially, informed consent, I argue that whilst these issues can be very important, these are only means to preserve human autonomy, dignity and safety, and should be seen in this light, not as ends in themselves. I further argue that far from being routinely excluded from most research designs, much greater effort should be made to include vulnerable populations and individuals, but with relevant safeguards. Comfortable notions of the existence of standard ethical issues with ready-made solutions are challenged, together with assumptions that certain concerns are a 'given' and not subject to negotiation and review.

Martin Johnson offers a novel perspective on undertaking ethical review of research in Chapter 6, an activity, to date, generally not included in published guidance and critique. He argues that the ability, and perhaps the motivation, to criticise constructively the work of others is far from well-developed in health and nursing research. Examples of the genre are rare, but with these he outlines questions that might be asked about research conduct and some of the issues that might need to be discussed. It needs to be remembered that critique is of the work, not the person, and should be taken in that light. We all make decisions in research that we might not recommend to others, and only through wider discussion of these can we begin to refine our approaches. Posing thirteen questions for the reviewer's attention, he illuminates the chapter with examples of studies that have been more or less rigorous in observing ethical standards. A risk–benefit approach is maintained together with a focus on assessing the justification for actions.

Research governance has become a major issue not only for the central authorities in the UK, but also for the many researchers who have struggled since its introduction to work through the additional bureaucracy of the new quality mechanisms. In Chapter 7 Michelle Howarth and Rosie Kneafsey recognise two sides to this conflict and provide a clear account of the essential features (incorporating comparisons with other countries), including the means to operationalise and implement such frameworks in practice. They present a very balanced account, noting the important benefits of the approach and keeping a lid on the irritation that they and almost all researchers endured when the bureaucracy behind these processes became, in many cases, out of all proportion to the incidences of harm it prevented, if any. As they note, progress is being made on the 'busting bureaucracy' front, but only time will tell if common sense prevails in most cases.

In Chapter 8, informed by her own service on an NHS Research Ethics Committee (REC), Carol Haigh gives practical advice on seeking formal approval. The rapidly changing format and processes of application for ethics approval under varying circumstances are explained, with clear illumination of the implications for the researcher. That approval by a NHS Research Ethics Committee may be less intimately linked to guarantees of ethical research than is often supposed is just one of the arguments featured in Carol Haigh's chapter on securing ethics approval. Unambiguous, practical advice on how to make a successful application is provided, together with clarification of the perspective of ethics committee members.

Chapter 9, by Debbie Fallon and Tony Long, offers an alternative to received wisdom about research ethics committees, suggesting that they are neither necessary nor the only means to ensure ethical conduct in research. Reviewing the reasons why RECs and current research governance arrangements may fail to provide an effective means to prevent unethical studies and to promote sound ethical research, we warn against the development of an era of passive ethical control that excuses the researcher from ethical responsibility, relying upon central systems of review, guidance and monitoring. We recommend the adoption, at least in certain aspects of research, of the social-science model of personal responsibility and peer review within a system of self-governance.

Intervention in research is the often-neglected subject of Martin Johnson's Chapter 10. Actions to meet participants' needs may be planned (as in 'hygienic' research) or on-the-spot and intuitive (as in 'messy' research). Research in the traditional scientific domain may provoke the paradox of being required to measure potential benefits and harms (and to state the respective intervention to be taken) before undertaking an intervention study yet needing the results of the study to be able to gauge these effects. An alternative dilemma is explored of when or whether to intervene to ensure safety or wellbeing of participants when the outcome of such action is unclear. The argument indicates the need to draw a line beyond which the risk to the subject or participant is too great and intervention is required, but the identification of this boundary is fraught with difficulty and requires serious consideration. The problems are found to be no easier in qualitative designs, although action research may provide a more ideal context in which to incorporate intervention within the study design. Drawing on feminist or situational ethics, an alternative strategy is suggested for messy research, available to all as a humanistic approach.

In the following Chapter 11 Carol Haigh and Neil Jones discuss what will be to many a mysterious world: that of Internet research. The potential of the Internet as a research medium is explored together with the significant concerns about the new risks associated with 'cyber research'. The Internet has an instantaneous and, to some extent, anonymous nature that makes it seem an ideal medium for cost-effective research. The pitfalls are many, however, and need to be fully explored by anyone thinking that this is a quick and easy route to data. A cyber-ethics framework is proposed to aid the techno-researcher in engaging in research using these novel means in the virtual world of cyberspace.

Finally, Martin Johnson uses Chapter 12 to debate issues relating to the dissemination of research findings: an area not normally considered in discussion of ethical conduct in research. Many research relationships end in acrimony (famously Barney Glaser and Anselm Strauss) in disputes over 'intellectual property', authorship or plagiarism. Careful negotiation and planning can reduce this risk. As regards ethics it seems that some journals will fail to publish work that was not approved by relevant ethics committees. Martin argues that simply insisting on that particular box being ticked will not guarantee that authors conducted their study to high standards. What is important is that ethical issues are discussed, in detail if necessary, and when things go wrong or were questionable, that this is offered for the research community to learn from. Ethical treatment of colleagues and fellow-researchers is considered as well as the means to provide adequate and convincing reassurance for the professional audience that the study to be reported was conducted in an ethically acceptable manner.

Our purpose in writing this book is to provide an easily available reference source that sets out in plain English important issues in the conduct of research from the point of view of maximising benefits and minimising harms. Research, as is the case with clinical judgement, needs to appeal to a risk-management framework in which important work will be conducted in balance with the needs of individuals and groups. We offer this through reasoned analysis and the presentation of alternative arguments in a manner that we hope will provide both clarification and stimulation to further analysis.

2

The individual in research

Tracey K Williamson

INTRODUCTION

In situations where participants in a study are simply research subjects, there are a number of ethical issues in need of consideration. Using an explicitly rights-based approach can help to clarify the issues explored here that involve the rights of participants as individuals or as members of groups. Involvement of service users in research as informants, co-researchers and user-researchers is also examined later in the chapter.

INDIVIDUALS' RIGHTS
Right to be informed

In most studies, participants need to appreciate fully what they are getting into in order that they can consent to participate prior to taking part. The situation for participants less than 18 years of age is somewhat different (Coyne 1998) and is described more fully in Chapter 4. A standard mechanism for the relaying of information about a study is the participant information sheet, which must have content that meets the requirements of the Central Office for Research Ethics Committees (COREC). However, in a study of information sheets used in research, many were found to exceed recommended reading levels, and researchers are encouraged to improve the readability of their documents (Franck & Winter 2004).

In studies with more of an emergent design, such as action research, it is not always possible to know what lies ahead, as such decisions are to be made in due course with participants. Information giving, checking of understanding, and assurances that consent to being involved is informed may need renegotiating at various points throughout the entire study. Health and social care researchers often undertake their research in settings that have a transient population. For example, in my own action research study of group decision-making in an NHS trust (Williamson 2004), new group members joined the groups being observed as part of the study. New participants had to be informed and their consent gained individually over the 3-year study period. Such an ongoing process to consent is well recognised amongst researchers employing participant-observation approaches (Merrell & Williams 1994).

When undertaking research with populations, such as community groups, or condition-specific groups such as stroke clubs, researchers need to be mindful of others in the vicinity of fieldwork. They need to have due regard for bystanders on the periphery who may not be a part of the study, but who are present in the setting (Moore & Savage 2002). Their presence raises issues about confidentiality not only in terms of what they may be privy to, but also in relation to information that may become evident concerning them as individuals as they go about their business in the research setting. Such situations arose in the above study where outside speakers attended meetings where decision-making processes were being observed. Their presence and actions could not be ignored as they interacted with the staff being studied, yet to inform and gain consent from them all would have been inappropriate. Instead, their actions were noted as contextual material, supplemented by the minutes of the meeting, but no direct reference was ever made to them in the study findings.

In a small number of studies, it is asserted that consent cannot be given beforehand as it would introduce bias to the results and so consent is gained retrospectively (Boter et al. 2004) with full approval from ethics committes in the researchers' own country (in Boter's case this was The Netherlands). Other acceptable reasons for not gaining consent include instances when people are unable to consent due to lack of capacity, for example when unconscious. Here proxy consent by a relative or other advocate may be appropriate.

Right to withdraw

Any individual has the right to withdraw from a study at any point, for whatever reason and they are not obliged to give a reason. They have the right not to have their care affected negatively or their relationships with the researchers, study funders or commissioners affected as a result of their withdrawal. Thus, the freely made choice to take part should be given to being rescinded just as easily. In any study, such withdrawal will be a disappointment to the researchers, who may have spent time and energy recruiting participants and undertaking the research. This raises issues about whether data already collected can be used (Meyer 1993). For example, in a study employing a series of interviews over time, data collected previously may be useable with the participant's permission even if they refuse to take part in subsequent interviews. In many studies, such as some trials, the data will be meaningless without completion of the study and so no decision about excluding or including data already collated need be made. It is up to the individual researcher to protect the rights of participants and act professionally whatever the consequences to their research. In some circumstances, if a participant is questioning their involvement, they may have fears that can be allayed or questions that can be answered, but under no circumstances must coercion be used to encourage continuation. It is usual for consent forms to make explicit the participants' right to withdraw without negative consequences.

Right not to be harmed

In any study there is potentially some degree of harm. Sometimes, the researcher may have to withdraw a participant from a study if it is in their best interests to do so. For example, in the case of a trial of a product, participants can expect that should an intervention be found conclusively not to work they should be prevented from enduring any more of the ineffective intervention. More recently, there has been a move to ensure that participants continue to receive an intervention after a study has finished if it is found to work well for them. On other occasions distress may be caused by the topic itself or simply as a result of asking people general questions about their experiences. In a study eliciting patients' views of the nurse clinician role (Williamson 2001), a small number of medical ward in-patient participants were tearful at the outset of their qualitative interview simply through being asked to describe their hospital stay so far. As is not uncommon, with reassurance and an offer to stop the interview or pause, participants chose to continue, keen to share their experiences, explaining their upset away as general anxiety incurred by hospital admission. Topics need not be overtly sensitive in order to result in mild upset. Great care is needed when topics are obviously sensitive, such as experiences of road traffic accidents or miscarriage. The potential difficulties in these situations can usually be managed satisfactorily by appropriate research techniques, such as using a skilled interviewer or careful questionnaire design.

Discomfort or harm do not necessarily occur at the time of the research activity and so strategies need to be in place to deal with these should they present. Contact details of someone who can give further information or support are usually to be found in participant information documents with help-line information or access to counsellors also being available in some instances. All participants should be informed of the right to complain, and the mechanism to do so should be clear to respondents in the event of researcher negligence. A participant's general practitioner should also be informed with their permission where the research may have an impact on the medical management of their physical or mental wellbeing.

Right to be researched

It is true to say that particular groups of the general population are more likely to be involved in research either intentionally or unintentionally. For example, limited resources, lack of access to interpreting services or concerns about the validity of tools, such as questionnaires if subjected to translation, means that English-speaking individuals with a certain degree of literacy tend to be more readily recruited across a range of studies. Some researchers are better than others at optimising inclusion so that, where appropriate to the study design, a greater cross section of possible participants is recruited. For example, studies of adults with diabetes will need to respect the larger numbers of people from Asian communities who have diabetes, and so every effort should be made to make recruitment materials available to non-English speakers. It is good ethical practice to give opportunity for involvement to anyone who is suitable and not to rule people's participation out by using methods or materials that are inaccessible to them. In some cases certain groups have been excluded for good reason. For example, with women there may be concerns about fertility and risk to any unborn child. However, women have sometimes been inappropriately excluded from study despite the often important influence of gender on results. Usefully, guidance has been produced to optimise women's involvement in research where it is appropriate (National Committee for Medical Research Ethics in Norway 2001).

In the UK, health and social care policy and research funders' interests have led to a number of priorities for research being identified. These include coronary heart disease, stroke, cancer, child health and mental health (Department of Health (DH) 2000). As a consequence, considerable funding is allocated to research in these areas and so certain groups of people have become very attractive target populations for researchers. Contrastingly, other funders, such as the Leverhulme Trust, have set out to fund studies that do not fit neatly into the traditional boundaries of other funding agencies. Whilst people have the right to be involved in research, the reality is that resource constraints and preferences for certain research topics by those who fund or commission research prevent some people from doing so.

There are a number of ways that potential participants can be purposefully excluded. Local Research Ethics Committees (LRECs) are mindful of this and ask researchers directly for any exclusion criteria, partly to protect participants by ensuring that some are excluded for their own good, such as people with severe heart disease not being recruited to a study involving extreme exercise. Pregnant women are often excluded from research interventions that may put their unborn child at risk, such as in studies involving X-rays. A problem arises when people or groups are excluded for no good reason, such as older people or those with a terminal illness. These groups are often excluded by researchers out of a misplaced wish to avoid inconvenience to them. Whilst it is important that participants have the capacity to participate, individuals or groups should not be ruled out as a result of discrimination. Not only would these people miss out on the opportunity to be involved, but they would also be excluded from any potential benefits, such as a new treatment or personal satisfaction of contributing to a greater understanding of the topic being investigated. They may already be considered disadvantaged as a result of their age or medical condition and then be disadvantaged again by not being included (double jeopardy).

A balance needs to be struck between the needs of what can be considered potentially vulnerable groups of people (e.g. older people, children, terminally ill people, people with visual impairments and people with mental-health needs) and their right and ability to participate. At an LREC hearing, a study involving single interviews with people who had had a stroke was presented that indicated that people with dementia might be included. This was questioned by the committee, which later accepted that their inclusion was important so as not to discriminate against people who have been labelled with a particular diagnosis. Through discussion, committee members were reassured that individuals' capacity to consent would be considered on an individual basis, as having dementia did not necessarily mean that people were incapable of offering informed consent and participating fully. Of course, what the committee was really concerned with was whether the investigator appreciated and could manage these issues. This was shown to be the case and the study was approved. Other researchers have adapted methods aimed at best engaging particular participants and meeting their perceived needs. For example, Curtis et al. (2004) undertook a study of children's views of health services, which used interviews, play and a website, and included 'hard-to-reach' children, such as asylum seekers and those with learning difficulties.

Right not to be over-researched

A further ethical concern is the over-researching of some populations, such as clients of infectious diseases and cancer services. Interestingly, some of the groups prioritized for research have claimed they have been 'researched to death' in recent years as illuminated by a study with black and ethnic-minority older people (Butt & O'Neil 2004). As part of ethical review processes, researchers are required to note participants' previous involvement in research so as not to exhaust certain social groups and to encourage involvement of other people not already involved in a study. In some instances, potentially vulnerable participants, such as those with a terminal illness may want to be involved in several or a succession of studies, which they may consider to constitute their last hope. The key is not to over-research individuals, yet have regard for their wishes and for any implications of their being in more than one study simultaneously.

Those individuals who do take part in a study should be able to expect not to be overtaxed by it. Sometimes researchers are over-zealous about what is reasonable for a participant to endure, including combinations of physical tests, such as exercise tolerance, large batteries of time-consuming questionnaires, and daily diaries to complete in addition to being interviewed. Essentially, information provided to potential participants should set out these requirements so that each individual can make their own mind up. However, LRECs have been known to challenge studies where excessive work or endurance is indicated. On occasion, researchers have split a proposed study into two to minimise the exertion required of participants. This suggests that, at times, the research community has proposed studies that are onerous rather than apply for separate approvals for two smaller more manageable studies in the first place.

Right to payment

There is no automatic right to receive payment or to benefit directly from participation in a study. It is common practice for participants to be made aware that, whilst they may not benefit personally from their involvement, the study findings may benefit others and so they may consent to take part for altruistic reasons (Smith 2003). Thus, the study findings may inform practices used with future users of health and social care services to their advantage. Some people do benefit, although that cannot be guaranteed, and information given to participants must not raise unrealistic expectations. For example, in a randomised controlled trial of a medication or treatment, participants need to be clear that they may not be allocated to the intervention arm and even if they were, that there would be no guarantee that the treatment being tested works any better than usual care.

What is common in certain types of studies, such as those recruiting students, is to offer payment to offset any inconvenience incurred by taking part. So long as the amount offered is appropriately modest, reflecting the amount of inconvenience that is likely, then there is no ethical problem. However, payment does become a problem if it is at a level that can be construed as excessive simply to recruit people, especially if the participants would endure some discomfort or be particularly taxed by involvement. Arguably, the temptation might be for people from less well-off backgrounds to participate for financial gain and thus be manipulated to participate. Nevertheless, whatever an individual's social background, they still have the right to decide for themselves what is reasonable.

In some studies of a participatory nature, it has been possible to make payments to participants acting as co-researchers for their time, often in the form of shopping vouchers or, less commonly, monetary payment. Why should people not be paid appropriately for work often undertaken in their own time? Unfortunately, funders who acknowledge the need for proper recompense are few and far between. Even less common are funders and commissioners who appreciate the amount of time that involving people as co-researchers in studies can take and so this aspect of research continues to be poorly resourced. The issue of payments remains an ongoing problem as there are implications for some participants who receive social security benefits and there are limits to what people can 'earn' without those benefits being affected or, at worst, withdrawn. Advice and accepted benefits practice varies from locality to locality. INVOLVE (2003) provides a useful source of guidance for good practice concerning payments to research participants.

Rights of ownership

Ownership involves two key issues: the data produced within a study and any bodily samples. In terms of ownership of the data, this would normally belong to the researcher; however, in studies that have a co-researcher relationship, such as participatory studies, this is less clear as they too may have some claim to the data. Similarly, the source of the funding for a study will also have implications, such as when an outside researcher is commissioned to undertake research within an organisation. These issues are explored further in Chapter 12 under authorship rights. In relation to the issue of samples such as blood specimens, this is commonly navigated by careful phrasing study information sheets and consent forms indicating that samples are provided as a gift for future research, with the specific nature of the research clearly specified.

Right to confidentiality and anonymity

Details about participants' involvement should be kept in confidence by the research team. This includes their personal information, such as contact details and any other identifiable material. LREC applications require individuals who will be privy to participants' information to be named. Those permitted are usually the researcher, research-team members, any supervisor in the event of the study being primarily part of an education programme, such as a Masters degree, and any administrators, such as those transcribing tape recorded interviews. Sharing of data is kept to a minimum and to people who have a professional responsibility to maintain confidentiality. In studies that involve lay people as co-researchers, particular arrangements need to be checked out with the appropriate research and development departments from the organisations where the research is to take place.

Participants need to be clear about the distinct difference between anonymity and confidentiality. Data will often be shared in a condensed form or as direct participant quotes from questionnaires or interviews, yet normally these will have been anonymised so that the participant cannot be recognised from these or any presentation of the study findings. In cases where this is difficult, it is good practice to ask the participant's permission prior to using their material. An example of this might be that when referring to findings from a small group of people, they might be recognisable by the choice of words used in the extract selected from the transcription or by job titles. Many organisations will have requirements around the divulgence of their identity depending on what the findings say about their staff or their services and where the findings are being presented. For example, it is not uncommon for NHS trusts to wish to remain anonymous by being referred to as 'a large non-teaching hospital in the North West of England' and so on. In using direct quotations, reference to pseudonyms or codes (e.g. Participant 4) is usual practice (see Chapter 12).

Confidentiality can be difficult to maintain in studies where the researcher is internal to the organisation or group they are researching. Role blurring may occur as one minute the researcher is an investigator and the next minute a senior member of staff in the researched organisation, interacting with the same people (Williamson 2004). A further difficulty relates to knowing which information is divulged in a research context and which information is offered in a non-research context. As Punch (1986) explains, there is a lack of distinction between what is public and what is private and so the way around this is to ensure confidentiality. In my study of shared governance (Williamson 2004), I clarified any uncertainty about the use of information with the participants at an appropriate point in the encounter or simply did not record the information in question. However, this is not always easy to do and it is acknowledged that information cannot always be disregarded if already committed to memory and it may colour future interpretations or actions. Another tactic I used was to discuss issues of confidentiality and anonymity with participants to gain their view of what was acceptable and to verify their understanding of the issues, particularly as they relaxed and divulged more freely over the passage of time. On occasion, occurrences of a sensitive nature took place, such as disagreement between individuals. Participants were assured that these events would be treated with discretion and tact, which they accepted. I refrained from writing notes about these incidents in detail, preferring to note them mentally instead. Individuals on the periphery who came into the research setting, yet were not being personally researched, were referred to loosely in field notes to protect their anonymity, for example, as a 'member of academic staff from a local university'.

It is usual that participant identifiable data are anonymised at the first opportunity by the researcher or by the custodian of the data, such as an administrator in charge of a database from which information is being made available. This includes name, address and postcode as a minimum and may also mean data, such as date of birth and record number (e.g. NHS/hospital records number). In most studies there is no requirement to be able to link research data with the participant it originated from and, therefore, data can be truly anonymous. In some cases, where a change in treatment or a diagnosis may be identified, the partial anonymity can be undone by cross-referencing coded data with a list of participants, usually kept separate and safeguarded strictly to prevent unauthorised linking of data to participant. LRECs will not permit, without good reason, designs that make these linkages possible and will insist on complete anonymity where appropriate. It is therefore important to make issues around the degree of anonymity and confidentiality clear to potential participants in study information sheets.

Rights of the researcher

A further point to stress is the right of a researcher or contributor to a study, such as a data inputter, to withdraw their participation should it become ethically unsound to continue. It is common to assist colleagues by collecting or inputting for their studies. Rarely, you may be asked to undertake tasks that are inappropriate, such as inventing data to complete gaps in data sets, or manipulating the data to be more favourable, such as adjusting records of response times when evaluating the effectiveness of a service. In these instances, everyone needs to be aware of the consequences of their actions in terms of their employment, potential harm to patients, integrity of the research community, research and clinical governance requirements, and public confidence. It is usual for organisations to have 'whistle-blowing' policies for researchers and others to make use of in these situations.

As well as participants, researchers' exposure to potential harm should be minimised. Risks present in a number of ways and commonly involve the researchers' safety when undertaking fieldwork. For example, when visiting the home of a participant, the person being visited may not be known to the researcher making it difficult for them to make a judgement about the risk to themself. Even where a participant is known to the researcher, there will be a chance that something could go badly wrong, such as the participant becoming upset and aggressive, or, indeed, the presence of another party or a pet may pose a threat. Similar issues are presented when undertaking fieldwork with groups often in premises that are unfamiliar to the researcher. These need not necessarily be well-recognised, high-risk settings, such as mental-health secure units, which need their own careful risk-management assessment and strategies. Risk can occur anywhere and so researchers need to take steps to be suitably familiar with their surroundings and escape routes in the event of fire or other urgent situations, and they should adopt good practices. These include the use of mobile phones to ring in to a colleague, action plans in the event of a researcher failing to make contact, or the presence of a companion in certain situations. Establishments that regularly undertake research usually have fieldwork guidelines to follow, whereas community settings, health visiting, for example, tend to have their own procedures, such as lone worker policies.

Care needs to be taken in terms of what information is divulged to research participants that may come back to harm the researcher in a number of ways. A simple example is for researchers not to give out their home addresses or personal home or mobile phone numbers. This may seem obvious, but studies have presented for ethical review with those exact mistakes. Relationships with participants may not remain amicable and, such information can be abused later. A significant number of studies are by researchers who have insight into the topic under study, for example, ex-mental-health service users investigating depression. Whilst rapport may need to be built for the purposes of the research, as when putting a participant at ease, too much sharing of personal information by the researcher about their experiences may not bode well for the relationship dynamics. Emotional involvement is a real possibility especially with longitudinal studies where familiarity and friendships may develop over time. Leaving the field is a well recognised challenge, especially in qualitative research (Morse & Field 1996). Bringing closure to a study can be a significant wrench for either party, perhaps managed best by making a gradual withdrawal yet with a clear endpoint being arrived at.

USER INVOLVEMENT IN RESEARCH

In the previous section, individuals as participants tended to be on the receiving end of a study's processes. What follows is explanation of what is meant by the term 'user involvement' so that it can be distinguished from participation in research as 'the researched'.

Background

Involvement of users of services and their carers in decisions about their care and development of health and social care services is of growing importance. Findings from the National Listening Exercise (National Co-ordinating Centre for NHS Service Delivery and Organisation (NCCSDO) 2000) indicate the significance that users place upon involvement in such service planning, as all too often inaccurate assumptions are made by professionals as to the needs and preferences of the public. User involvement in all stages of the research process is similarly a government priority (Calnan & Gabe 2001). This is reflected in a range of government and other publications that have an emphasis on involving those who are current or potential recipients of health and social care in its development (DH 2004, Royal College of Nursing 2004). The need to ensure that research addresses the topics of concern and importance to the public is made explicit in policy that demands their involvement in all stages of the research process (DH 2000).

There has been a shift amongst research funders, with many now requiring user involvement to be demonstrated within funding applications (O'Donnell & Entwistle 2004a). For several years now the Department of Health has funded an advisory group, known as INVOLVE, whose remit is to promote public and patient involvement in health and social care, and public-health research. Furthermore, a number of groups with an interest in promoting and supporting users' involvement in research have also emerged (e.g. North West Users Research Advisory Group, Service Users Research Group for England (SURGE)). Correspondingly, those who appraise research applications, such as research and development departments and LRECs, are required to gain the views of lay representatives as part of their review processes. However, recognising a value in having user involvement does not necessarily translate into that involvement being secured, either at all or in a meaningful way. Even where involvement does take place in research studies, authors infrequently write about it in their publications (Chambers et al. 2004). Plainly, user involvement in research is subject to a number of ethical challenges to be managed. I will now explore these ethical tensions and ways of dealing with them.

Defining user involvement

As a leading authority on user involvement in research, INVOLVE (2004) provides the following definition:

An active partnership between the public and researchers in the research process, rather than the use of people as the 'subjects' of research. Active involvement may take the form of consultation, collaboration or user control. Many people define public involvement in research as doing research 'with' or 'by' the public, rather than 'to', 'about' or 'for' the public .

(INVOLVE 2004).

The phrase 'involving users in research' can be misleading, as those who may be involved originate from across the spectrum of the general public. INVOLVE (2004) has expanded on the term 'public' to include the following:

- Consumers
- Patients and potential patients
- People who use health and social services
- Informal (unpaid) carers and parents
- Members of the public who may be targeted by health-promotion programmes
- Organisations that represent the public's interests
- Communities that are affected by public-health or health- and social-care issues
- Groups asking for research because they believe they have been exposed to potentially harmful substances or products (e.g. pesticides or asbestos).

For convenience, the overarching term 'user' will be used from this point to embrace all of the above terms.

Research 'with' or 'on'

Involving users as mere subjects or participants within a research study is not what is intended by advocates of involvement. Whilst studies such as some clinical trials comprise research 'on' people, others adopt the approach of research 'with' people, yet each has possibilities for user involvement. Certainly, some types of study may lend themselves more readily to user involvement. Yet even those that at first may appear unsuited have significant potential for meaningful involvement. Recognition that users can play a more active part in research is not new. Their involvement is known to pay dividends in terms of consulting with their peers and prioritising research topics (Oliver et al. 2004), although the ways in which their input is sought influences the impact that they have. For example, the decision-making structures and processes in place, types of users, timing of their input and methods for contributing have been found to moderate the effect users can have on a study (O'Donnell & Entwistle 2004b).

A range of research approaches encourages, indeed necessitates, the involvement of users as co-researchers in ways that represent an active partnership between users and the research team. The latter often comprises professional (academic or practitioner) researchers. A good example of successful collaborative working is a study by Rose et al. (2003) in which service-user researchers and academic researchers worked together in partnership to explore perceptions of electro-convulsive therapy. What is becoming increasingly common in recent years is research that is user-led and even user-controlled. The difference between these is the emphasis of the latter on users being in full control, whereas user-led research 'may be funded from within an organisation where some control is retained but is led by service users' (Faulkner 2005). For example, Faulkner and Layzell (2000) report on a study of mental-health service users' experiences of therapy and treatment for their mental-health needs that was conceived, designed and undertaken entirely by service users.

Degrees of involvement

Involvement can be realised in a number of guises and to varying extents. A common way of looking at involvement is as a range from full participation in all activities and decision making, to merely being kept informed. In research terms, points along the spectrum may include 'consultation' on drafts or ideas, acting as 'informants' such as at study-design developmental workshops, acting in partnership as 'co-researchers' and through to the role of lead researchers as in user-led and user-controlled studies. The extent of involvement may be pre-determined by the professional researchers or depending on the type of study, it may be put to users to decide the extent of their involvement. Ways of being involved may differ from user to user depending on their skills or interests and also at certain points in time. Users may like to be involved in interview-guide development, but not in interviewing itself, or may have more time on their hands at certain times of the year. A useful tactic is to employ some means of ascertaining users' preferences, previous skills, knowledge and interests, networks and contacts, and expectations, so as to get the most out of their input. The key is to avoid tokenism and embrace the valuable contribution that many users can make.

Reasons for involving users in research

The added value of involving users in research is potentially far reaching:

- **Design**. Asking users to comment on proposed study design or draft tools or participate fully in design discussions can lead to a more appropriate design being finalised. For the researchers and funders, this may increase the likelihood of a well-executed study in return for their investments of time and money. Studies underpinned by poor science and findings that lack meaning are unethical if they risk not reaching a standard that makes the work worthwhile, particularly where public money is being spent. Greater involvement in designing studies and tools *with* users can further enhance their validity by ensuring the right questions are asked and phrased in the right way. The researching organisation may also gain credibility by involving users.
- **Recruitment**. Users may well have insights that can lead to better plans for sampling and recruitment to a study through their existing knowledge of the topic, contacts, networks and links and appreciation of which ways of approaching people may work best. Their views on choices of recruitment media, wording and where, when and how to circulate recruitment materials can be very helpful. This was certainly the case in a study of loneliness amongst older people, which aimed to identify strategies older people use to prevent and deal with loneliness and isolation (University of Salford/Age Concern Wigan 2005). Older people trained as co-researchers were actively involved in devising a sampling frame, recruitment materials and a distribution plan. Their involvement met with considerable success in reaching older people at the places that they frequent and in ways that appeal to them.
- **Hard to reach groups**. Groups to which it is difficult to gain access, such as people with a visual impairment or from certain ethnic backgrounds, present challenges to researchers particularly if they themselves are seen to have little in common with potential participants. These so-called 'hard-to-reach' groups are those who may lack structures of representation, may have difficulty meeting with service user representatives and managers, or are subject to attitudes and legislation that hinder their involvement in development of health and social care services (NCCSDO 2003). Minority

groups cited by the NCCSDO include carers, young people, older people, black people, people of ethnic-minority background, travellers, the homeless and those with learning difficulties. Thus, an 'insider' perspective can be valuable in securing access and in ensuring appropriate behaviour once inside groups, organisations or in meetings with individuals. Not to do so can again lead to poorly constructed study design and less meaningful results. In this context, findings that lack relevance to the current or future population that they concern can be considered unethical.

- **Dissemination.** If research is worth doing it is worth disseminating. Strategies for reaching those involved in research as researched, co-researchers or informants with study findings are generally considered ethically important as reflected in LREC application requirements. Nonetheless, this can be a neglected part of the research process as pressures to complete studies within timeframes and funding limits can lead to hurried dissemination activities. Involvement of users can help to identify where to disseminate to reach user audiences, what format and media to disseminate in, and even assist with dissemination, whether it is distribution of findings summaries; writing for newsletters or publications; or presenting at clubs, networks and conferences. Thus, equity can be achieved by disseminating beyond 'professional' audiences and by fulfilling participants' right to know the outcome of their involvement (see Chapter 12).

- **Personal benefits.** Users may personally benefit in a variety of ways including increased confidence, a sense of making a difference, acquisition of new skills, social opportunities and by developing their existing or future career pathways. All these are positive outcomes that can be enhanced with careful thought by researchers. It is worth considering whether users' expectations should be viewed as any less important than our own as researchers. Whilst it is helpful to keep some degree of organisation when meeting and working with users, it is equally important to build in time to socialise or for discussions to go off track a little. In another study (Williamson 2005) research design meetings with users occasionally went off at a tangent as they recounted their experiences, for example of hospital or social care, or when they did not conform with the way professionally dominated meetings are conducted. Whilst not advocating chaos, there are good reasons to ensure users' personal needs are met from any research encounter, such as making time for them to bring their own topics to the discussion. Many will be there in their own time, with little or no payment in financial terms and so seek other 'benefits'. Often it will be down to the personal ethics of the research team as to how such ways of working are managed.

- **_Ownership_**. Particularly in studies adopting an empowering approach, involvement of people in matters that concern them can lead to them taking some responsibility for addressing the problem, commitment to seeking solutions and then ownership of the outcomes.

Good practice for involvement

Involving users presents researchers with opportunities for creativity. There are existing resources providing guidance for general user involvement (City Hospitals Sunderland NHS Trust 2004) and these principles are directly transferable to user involvement in research. Various guides on user involvement in research are available through INVOLVE. Specific strategies include:

- Where possible, engage with users prior to the research project being initiated to build relationships and agree priorities for research
- Involve users as early as possible in the clarifying of an idea, formulation of a design, and preferred means of subsequent involvement, ensuring that this is not tokenistic
- Identify users' skills, knowledge, and previous experiences so that good use can be made of these
- Identify users' training and development needs and address these in ways that are accessible to them
- Identify users' support needs, such as a 'buddy' system, to help them navigate research activities and meetings
- Make sure meeting places are accessible in terms of location, times, mobility needs, acoustics, comfort, transport
- Use appropriate communication materials considering types of media, type font, who the audience is
- Develop research materials and tools with users and do not reject their suggestions out of hand
- Manage meetings to ensure the user's voice is heard and that other professionals conduct themselves appropriately, e.g. avoiding jargon
- Allow time for discussion and socialising
- Ensure user involvement embraces ethical principles in your own and others' practice.

In this chapter I have highlighted a range of ethical tensions to be managed in studies involving individuals or groups as research participants. I illustrate the scope of participation and involvement from being the researched to user-controlled research. Methods for involving people are many and it is up to researchers to be aware of the potential for unethical practices, to appreciate the value of involvement, and to explore ways of optimising meaningful involvement in research. Whilst involvement is an ongoing and fluid process, the recommendation is clearly to involve users and other stakeholders as early as possible in any research endeavour and, wherever possible, to build up relationships with users beforehand.

REFERENCES

Boter H, van Delden JJM, de Haan RJ, Rinkel GJE (2004) Patients' evaluation of informed consent to postponed information: cohort study. British Medical Journal 329, 86–87.

Butt J, O'Neil A (2004) "Let's move on": Black and minority ethnic older people's views on research findings. Joseph Rowntree Foundation.

Calnan M, Gabe J (2001) From consumerism to partnership? Britain's National Health Service at the turn of the century. International Journal of Health Services 31(1), 119–131.

Chambers R, O'Brian L, Linnell S, Sharp S (2004) Why don't health researchers report consumer involvement? Quality in Primary Care 12(2), 151–157.

City Hospitals Sunderland NHS Trust (2004) Patient involvement toolkit. CHSNT, Sunderland.

Coyne I (1998) Researching children: some methodological and ethical considerations. Journal of Clinical Nursing 7, 409–416.

Curtis K, Liabo K, Roberts H, Barker M (2004) Consulted but not heard: a qualitative study of young people's views of their local health service. Health Expectations 7, 149–156.

Department of Health (2000) Research and development for a first class service – R&D funding in the new NHS. HMSO, London.

Department of Health (2004) National service framework for children, young people and maternity services. HMSO, London.

Faulkner A (2005) Guidance for good practice. Service user involvement in the UK Mental Health Research Network. Service User Research Group, England.

Faulkner A, Layzell S (2000) Strategies for Living: a report of user-led research into people's strategies for living with mental distress. Mental Health Foundation, London.

Franck L, Winter I (2004) Research participant information sheets are difficult to read. Bulletin of Medical Ethics February 2004, 13–16.

INVOLVE (2003) A guide to paying members of the public who are actively involved in research: For researchers and research commissioners, (who may also be people who use services). INVOLVE: Hampshire.

INVOLVE (2004) http://www.invo.org.uk/About_Us.asp (accessed 01/08/05)

Merrell J, Williams A (1994) Participant observation and informed consent: relationships and tactical decision making in nursing research. Nursing Ethics 1(3), 163–172.

Meyer J (1993) New paradigm research in practice: the trials and tribulations of action research. Journal of Advanced Nursing 18, 1066–1072.

Moore L, Savage J (2002) Participant observation, informed consent and ethical approval. Nurse Researcher 9(4), 758–769.

Morse J, Field P (1996) Nursing Research. The application of qualitative approaches (Second Edition). Chapman and Hall: London.

National Committee for Medical Research Ethics in Norway (2001) Guidelines for the inclusion of women in medical research – gender as a variable in all medical research. http://etikkom.no/Engelsk (Accessed 01/08/05).

National Co-ordinating Centre for NHS Service Delivery and Organisation (2000) National listening exercise: report of the findings. NCCSDO: London.

National Co-ordinating Centre for NHS Service Delivery and Organisation (2003) User involvement in change management: A review of the literature. NCCSDO: London.

O'Donnell M, Entwistle V (2004a) Consumer involvement in research projects: the activities of research funders. Health Policy 69, 229–238.

O'Donnell M, Entwistle V (2004b) Consumer involvement in decisions about what health-related research is funded. Health Policy 70, 281–290.

Oliver S, Clarke-Jones L, Rees R et al. (2004) Involving consumers in research and development agenda setting for the NHS: developing an evidence based approach. Health Technology Assessment 8(15).

Punch M (1986) The politics of fieldwork. Qualitative Research Methods 3, Sage Publications, London.

Rose D, Wykes T, Leese M, Bindman J, Fleischmann P (2003) Patients' perspectives on electroconvulsive therapy: systematic review. British Medical Journal 326, 1363–1366.

Royal College of Nursing (2004) Caring in partnership: older people and nursing staff working towards the future. RCN, London.

Smith A (2003) Informed consent does not exist. The 2003 Ethics Forum Debate. Clinical Research Focus 14(5), 18–22.

University of Salford/Age Concern Wigan (2005) 'Saying Hello Each Day': combating loneliness and isolation amongst older people in Wigan. Working Paper 6: Research Design. University of Salford.

Williamson TK (2001) The roles and functions of the clinical nurse practitioner: patient and clinical nurse practitioner perspectives. Unpublished MSc dissertation: Liverpool John Moores University.

Williamson TK (2004) Strengthening decision-making within shared governance: an action research study. Unpublished PhD thesis. University of Salford.

Williamson TK (2005) Evaluation of a nurse led unit: an action research study. Research Design Workshop Reports 1-5. University of Salford.

USEFUL WEBSITES

INVOLVE (formerly Consumers in NHS Research) (accessed 01/08/05)
http://www.invo.org.uk
Research & Development North West (R&DNoW) (Host of North West Users Research Advisory Group) (Accessed 01/08/05)
http://www.lancs.ac.uk/fss/ihr/hrdn/userinvolvement.htm
Service User Research Group England (SURGE) (Accessed 01/08/05)
http://www.mhrn.info/surge.html
The Leverhulme Trust (Accessed 01/08/05)
http://www.leverhulme.org.uk

The theoretical and social context of research ethics

Martin Johnson

INTRODUCTION

Many research textbooks explain research methods and their ethical aspects as logical processes that follow a given number of steps. Research, however, does not take place in a vacuum. It is imagined, designed, planned, funded (or not), executed and reported in a complex social world by and with people with a whole range of viewpoints, values, needs, beliefs and agendas. In this chapter I will introduce some aspects of this complexity, particularly the social and theoretical context of research ethics.

THE SOCIAL CONTEXT OF RESEARCH ETHICS
Professional socialisation

The end of the Nazis in 1945 is commonly seen as the watershed in health research ethics, when experimentation by doctors and others that caused harms and death, it was believed, came to an end. Sadly, this is not so. Several countries have reported scientific fraud or seriously harmful conduct in medical fields since then. At about the time some of the first critiques of medicine and health care were being published (Freidson 1970), Beecher (1966), himself a professor of anaesthetics, demonstrated that Western medical scientists had published many gravely questionable studies. For example:

> During a (routine) bronchoscopy a special needle was inserted through a bronchus into the left atrium of the heart. This was done in an unspecified number of subjects, both with cardiac disease and with normal hearts.
>
> The technic[1] was a new approach whose hazards were at the beginning quite unknown. The subjects with normal hearts

---

[1] Beecher's spelling

were used, not for their possible benefit but for that of patients in general.

(Beecher 1966)

Giving a number of examples, Beecher notes that he has only sampled from the large amount of problematic research available at that time. Using the relevant death rates from the experimental procedures that had been tried without subjects' consent, Beecher shows that both suffering and death were certainly experienced in a large number of cases. We might ask, then, how it was that idealistic young health professionals wanting to relieve suffering and prevent death could be led into such approaches.

Health professionals in general, and nurses and doctors in particular, have always been of great interest to sociologists. They have been investigated, arguably, more than the clients and patients they serve. Studies of the passage of students through medical schools into practice and beyond demonstrate a change in the idealism so evident on entry, towards cynicism and pragmatism. Becker et al. (1961) called this the 'fate of idealism'. They argued that achievement in the profession meant examination success and mimicking the authoritarian and paternalistic behaviour of very senior doctors. This led to the loss of the initially more altruistic orientation. Similar changes were demonstrated in student nurses (Psathas 1968) and were widely perceived to be endemic to these occupations.

A good deal is known, therefore, about the ways in which health professionals come to learn their place in the health care hierarchy. We know, for example, that whatever students are taught in classes, it is the reality of clinical experience where the 'rules' are really learned. In the USA, Kramer (1974) brought attention to the difference between the managerial or bureaucratic values of the health care system and the professional values that students had been taught in the schools of nursing. The anxiety provoked by conflict of these different values as experienced by new graduates she termed 'reality shock'.

Studies of occupational socialisation in the UK (Melia 1987) have shown parallel outcomes, illustrating the difficulties of translating taught ideals, whether theory- or research-based evidence (Lacey 1994, Newell 2002), into day-to-day practice. This also means that we cannot assume that by teaching codes of research conduct and ethical theories to neophyte health professionals they will behave in all matters with patients' interests uppermost in their mind.

A right to investigate?

The extremely paternalistic and thoughtless attitudes illustrated by Beecher were not confined to physicians and surgeons, although the dangers they are able to create for research participants are, arguably, greater than most. By keeping details of their car registrations, sociologist Humphreys (1975) probably risked revealing the identity of many of the gay men he secretly studied in (then, as now, illegal) sex acts mainly in public toilets (see Chapter 5), and Field (1989) reported work done covertly by his research student to study the care of people dying in hospital wards. Even in the 1980s Field, in particular, was merely using the norms of the time, in which the covert observation and recording of social life were seen as the natural work of the sociologist, because more open study might lead to behaviour not being 'natural and normal'.

Whilst for 100 years medicine was seen as the 'academic base' of nursing and the 'professions allied to medicine', increasingly some of these subordinate professions have looked to sociology and anthropology for their models of research conduct. The influence of grounded theory and related interpretive approaches on nursing research has been profound, but investigators in these traditions have sometimes seen the need for ethical approval or informed consent for research participants as either unnecessary or obstructive to the pursuit of truth in a particular case (Clarke 1996, Field 1989).

As we can see, some research is undertaken without anyone's knowledge and sometimes the arguments that this was both necessary and for the great benefit of many are compelling. Such investigation is often undertaken in order to reveal poor practice about which health professionals cannot, or will not, complain.

A 2005 BBC *Panorama* programme *Undercover Nurse* used the increasingly fashionable ploy of a hidden camera to reveal very poor care of older people:

> *People lay in excruciating pain because analgesia was not administered properly. Others were distressed because they had to wait hours to use the toilet, while some were left to sit in their own excreta. Patients unable to feed themselves were left hungry and thirsty. One woman died alone, un-noticed. The programme was truly distressing.*
>
> (Humm & Lehane 2005)

Whilst such programmes may not conform to the analytic rigour of a 'research study', the means to collect data (covert participant observation) and the intentions are largely the same. Of course, the consequences in terms of public appreciation of the problems revealed are, through the medium of prime-time television, far greater. In this respect, both benefits and any harms of the approach are greatly amplified.

The failure of advocacy

Commenting on the programme, Humm and Lehane (2005) ask why the nurses involved had not done something about the poor care or complained. They suggest that nurses are fearful of being branded as troublemakers and that their complaints will fall on deaf ears. Here, and elsewhere, it is clear that nurses feel disempowered from taking the necessary steps to improve care and challenge policies and inadequate resources. If this is so in respect of care, then it is likely to be so with research itself. The medically subordinate health professions (Freidson 1970) have a cultural lack of assertiveness, particularly well-demonstrated in nursing, but also evident in some ranks of even the medical profession. This leads equally to an inability, or unwillingness, to challenge the nature and conduct of treatment, care or research (DH 2001).

Social work practitioners in the UK have been particularly criticised for their inability to 'challenge' the practice of social and other care workers and health professionals (The Victoria Climbié Inquiry 2003). Barbour (1985) studied the occupational socialisation of social workers. She showed how, when problems arise, social workers learn to comply with the definition of the situation and any constraints applied by those in authority, whilst maintaining private reservations. Later, most undergo 'internalised adjustment' in which they not only comply, but come to believe that the constraints they are under are for the best. Barbour does not use these ideas uncritically, and is herself concerned that individuals often negotiate their own situation depending on a given context. Indeed, she draws on the powerful concept of 'moral career', used so effectively by Goffman (1968) to mean the regularly re-negotiated social reputation of the individual. By means of this idea we can see that by using various tactics, such as 'keeping your head down' on small matters (Johnson 1997), relatively subordinate health professionals and even patients can negotiate a more significant role in more important decisions. Unfortunately, others 'keep their heads down' consistently, even when the consequences for very vulnerable individuals are dire.

Professional power

I have referred to the growing critique of medical and other health and social care workers which has, to some extent, increased the accountability (by which I mean public answerability for actions) of these workers in general, and medicine in particular. This critique has been both academic (Freidson 1970, Illich 1976) and present in the serious investigations of practice and research conduct (DH 2001, The Victoria Climbié Inquiry 2003). One important effect of the Royal Liverpool Children's Inquiry Report (DH 2001) was the introduction of several more detailed levels of scrutiny of practical research with living humans, despite the main issue in that report being the inappropriate retention, without relatives' consent, of pathology specimens; partly for potential research purposes. This deeper level of scrutiny, for the most part on paper and in advance of the proposed study, still leaves aside the questions that arise in the daily conduct of a research project once approved.

The gaze

Despite this new bureaucracy of 'research governance', it would be wrong to assume that professional power is significantly weakened in day-to-day care, or in the negotiation of research opportunities with patients. I will illustrate the disempowerment of most patients by discussing just one key aspect, the extreme subjugation of the patient to the 'gaze' of the health professional, in the most intimate of respects. A large and recent qualitative study of 72 older people in the UK (Woolhead 2004) showed that patients' dignity is often violated by staff leaving people's bodies exposed. In one situation a person in a stroke rehabilitation unit said:

> *[I was] on the hoist and I used to say 'can I cover myself up' and they just pulled your nightie down over you but the back view was wide open to anybody.*

(Woolhead 2004)

This example seems to be universal, with an Australian study revealing similar issues.

Walsh and Kowanko (2002) undertook a small, but interesting, qualitative study of a group of patients and nurses in South Australia. They show that patients felt very bodily exposed and suffered considerable humiliation. One person complained of being dressed in an operation gown that flew open at the back. She explains how she felt being taken to the bathroom:

...They don't bother to do it up and you're sitting in this chair, your bottom going through the hole and you say to them, 'Well look cover me up, I don't want to go out like this......' and they (nurses) just say, 'Oh you're in a public hospital now.'..you're taken out in front of visitors, maintenance people, cleaners, doctors walking around...

(Walsh and Kowanko 2002)

In the context of the care of dying people, Lawton (2000) brilliantly describes, then carefully analyses, the de-personalising effects of 'unboundedness'. We become unbounded when bodily secretions and waste products become public. We deal with sneezing quite well, but when such outputs are from the pelvic regions the more embarrassed, even humiliated, we feel when these products become public.

Nurses, doctors and some other health professionals expect routine access to the relevant orifices, which may of course be clinically necessary. There is, however, a general lack of privacy in what outside of health care would be extremely private bodily functions. Together with the generally superior medical knowledge and access to data about the patient, this lack of privacy contributes to what Foucault (1991) calls the 'gaze', the continued and penetrating surveillance of the living body. As Foucault argues at length, this gaze is the principal means to professional power. Being subject to the gaze ensures that patients can never be equals in the so-called professional–client partnership, since professionals never are subject to the patients' gaze in respect of intimate aspects of their life. The disempowerment of patients in this and other respects, such as not really knowing which treatments are best, reduces their autonomy during the negotiation of treatments, care or research into these interventions. It is particularly ironic that rather than empowering patients, most research methods merely compound the 'gaze' by invading personal privacy in some respect to produce data for others to use and therefore adds to the surveillance (Johnson 2005).

Despite these aspects, it is also true that with the advent of better education, information sources such as the Internet, and a general commitment in health care to include patients in decisions to a greater extent, many patients feel much more empowered and consulted about both care and any research they may be involved in.

Culture, 'race' and gender

There is a great need to improve the capture of data about the experiences of the whole range of social groups involved in research. All too often researchers use a sample for their own convenience rather than to examine the needs of a multi-layered society. This alone can mean that the diversity of the population remains hidden in research reports. Even in those cases where researchers have made genuine efforts to capture the experiences of minority communities they can be hard to reach, through difference in values, customs and willingness to use the services through which they might be recruited (Long 2004). Gunaratnam (2003) and Long (2004) suggest that the investigation of the experiences of minority communities has great moral importance whilst challenging our common conceptions of the basic analytic categories.

At a common sense level we all know that predetermined social and demographic categories are flawed. In an early study of my own (Johnson 1983) I asked questions about ethnic origin and religion to which some Jewish respondents raised objections, not because the questions were badly worded for the time, but because to these respondents their Jewishness was to them more complicated than a tick in a box. One nurse in particular considered herself to be a white European atheist, but wanted, nevertheless, to express her Jewishness as an issue of history, even of solidarity, in a way my questionnaire did not permit. For her being Jewish was not a religion, nor was it her 'ethnic group'.

Gunaratnam (2003) uses quotation marks around the word 'race'. This is meant to convey the fluid and essentially contested nature of its meaning. Indeed, it seems that the principle she espouses is that the idea of race is virtually meaningless. She traces the use of racial and ethnic categories in research showing how they are neither 'natural' nor 'neutral', but are socially and historically produced and are heavy with political meaning (p.11).

Gunaratnam, however, acknowledges the difficulties that political correctness can produce. She points to what she calls a 'doubled' research practice, in which researchers need to work both *with* and *against* (her emphasis) racial and ethnic categories. By this she seems to mean that researchers can work with the inadequate racial and ethnic categories that are to hand, whilst also finding ways of identifying and disrupting the ways in which these same categories can 'essentialise' race and ethnicity (i.e. render them permanent).

Although Gunaratnam critically examines a good deal of research that has used such categories and gives excellent examples from her own research into the hospice experiences of minority ethnic people, she provides no easy tool kit with which we can describe the social world with concepts and categories, and which will be both analytically useful and politically correct.

For example, in the study of an urban population's access to health services it remains necessary to use analytically useful, if crude, categories to determine equity or access to services. The same is true of social class. Hardly any individual is comfortable with the social class the Census ascribes to them since our class is a matter of personal employment and salary, education, our parent's place in life, where and what type of accommodation we live in and, perhaps even more importantly, the values we hold. But in planning for thousands or millions of people, the concept of class becomes analytically useful. In this macroscopic context we have to rely to a large extent on fairly crude definitions of the 'race' 'culture', 'ethnic group' and 'social class' of any population.

Gender

Gender, too, is a major aspect of the social context of research. Whilst men have certainly been misused in a research context, there is no doubt whatsoever that women have been systematically excluded from scientific study (Gilligan 1982) from which they, as a group, might have benefited. Gilligan argued that by eliminating women from his research samples, the influential Lawrence Kohlberg had eliminated a 'care focus' from his 6-stage theory of moral reasoning.

Even more importantly, women have been systematically exploited as research subjects (Johnstone 1994). In New Zealand, the Report of the Cervical Cancer Inquiry in 1988 followed allegations of the unethical treatment of women with cervical cancer in experiments at the National Women's Hospital in Auckland. These experiments involved the withholding of treatment for cervical cancer from women diagnosed as having carcinoma-in-situ in order to demonstrate that carcinoma-in-situ was not pre-malignant (Cartwright 1988, Dew & Roorda 2001).

Herbert Green, the principal investigator had felt that the possible reduced fertility following the treatment of carcinoma-in-situ was not acceptable. His aim was to study the natural history of the untreated disease. The women were never told that they had not been treated and about 40 of these women developed invasive cancer due to the withholding of treatment (Dew & Roorda 2001).

Dew and Roorda identify the difficulties women may face in confronting such situations. In the case of one woman, making a complaint against her GP included the emotional trauma experienced during the disciplinary hearing when she faced a panel of professional men and was cross-examined by her GP's lawyer. She also incurred a lawyer's bill of over $1000 that was the excess above the costs granted by the Committee. The doctor on the other hand was censured but his name was suppressed (Dew & Roorda 2001).

In order to assist in the examination of the values and perspectives that can be brought to bear on research conduct, by way of an introduction I will now explore three main approaches. Other viewpoints exist, and each may coincide in the analysis of a particular study.

ETHICAL PERSPECTIVES

Whilst in textbooks moral theories or perspectives can seem daunting and complicated, the recent movement by some philosophers, such as Harris (1985), to apply careful thought to problems in health care without too much reference to obscure 'philosophy' is helpful. In practical terms, many of the differences between eminent philosophers are subtle from the viewpoint of the clinician or practical researcher. With apologies to those with more philosophical training, what follows is a brief theoretical overview of ideas that may be brought to bear on any study.

Human rights

The 'human rights' perspective has been prominent for more than 60 years since World War II, when it became clear that human beings had been tortured, mutilated and killed for 'scientific' purposes by both military and civilian health workers. It is not surprising that many codes of conduct grew up in an effort to prevent such abuses in the future (WMA 2005). These tended to emphasise the right of individuals to be consulted about issues that affect them in research. In practical terms this has meant a strong emphasis on 'informed consent' to research activity in which individuals are involved or affected. However, other 'rights' are evident in this approach, such as a right to privacy (Moskop et al. 2005), a right to confidentiality, a right to anonymity, the right not to be harmed and the right to 'considerate and respectful care' (Benjamin & Curtis 1981). Benjamin and Curtis go on to argue that, especially in the USA (but now increasingly in Europe), greater susceptibility to litigation inflated the pressure to protect these 'rights' of research participants.

The 'rights' perspective is underpinned theoretically by some sound and generally well-argued philosophy best exemplified by a principle enunciated by the otherwise rather inaccessible Immanuel Kant. Edwards (1996) explains Kant's view quoting the following:

> *Act in such a way that you always treat humanity, whether in thine own person or in that of any other, never simply as a means but always at the same time as an end.*
>
> (Edwards 1996)

Edwards deduces from this that human beings should be considered to be autonomous and respected as such. This is often said to mean that no human should ever be treated as a means to an end. The theory has a certain attraction. Of course we should not use people just for our own ends and it seems really laudable to give everyone 'inalienable rights' and then to preserve them. Many codes of conduct and texts on research ethics suggest exactly this (see Johnstone 1994). Evaluating studies from this perspective ought to be straightforward, since codes of conduct, 'principles' or criteria are more explicit within this approach. For example, if we take the view, commonly expressed, that all research participants should be fully informed that they have been included in a study, perhaps even signing a consent form, then the following influential studies will be found wanting:

> *Nursing the dying* (Field 1989), Routledge, London
> *Behind the screens* (Lawler 1991), Churchill Livingstone, Edinburgh
> *On being sane in insane places* (Rosenhan 1973), Science 179, 250–258
> *The tearoom trade* (Humphreys 1975), Aldine, Chicago.

All these researchers secretly collected sensitive data from people who had no idea that they were being studied.

Are 'rights' useful?

Among other rights, it is common to assert the duty of the researcher to avoid harming research participants, which follows logically from the right of respondents not to be harmed. For example, Neville and Haigh (2003) seem to think it possible to do no harm:

The principle of non-maleficence requires us to do no harm. This fundamental principle forms the bedrock of the Declaration of Helsinki and could arguably be the raison d`etre of ethics committees.

(Neville and Haigh 2003)

Although 'rights-based' approaches to research conduct and approval are common, the classic text by Polit and Hungler (1999) is different in its approach. They begin their discussion of the ethical context of research by emphasising non-maleficence, which they argue encompasses the maxim 'above all do no harm'. They go on to suggest that 'exposing research participants to experiences that result in serious or permanent harm is unacceptable' (p.134). Already we can see that their position is not absolute. They are concerned about *serious* or *permanent* harm rather than any harm at all. In the case of asking sensitive questions they point out that the psychological consequences of asking people about their personal views, weaknesses or fears may cause them to admit to aspects of themselves or things they would rather forget. Polit and Hungler make the point, not that such questions should be avoided, but that it is necessary to think carefully about the nature of such intrusion, about the phrasing of such questions and about the need for de-briefing afterwards.

They later draw attention to the need for a thoughtful analysis by those involved of the benefits that may result from the investigation in balance with its risks. This risk–benefit approach can seem to deny the 'inalienable rights' such as not to be harmed, not to have privacy invaded and to be fully informed about all aspects of a study.

However, everything we do in life is a risk–benefit calculation, however deliberately or unconsciously worked out. Getting into the car, flying to conferences, having hip operations, taking medicines and 'doing nursing research' all risk harm. Harms are everywhere, as with the pain and risks of hip operations, so with poor questionnaires or insensitive interviewers, but there is a considerable difference in degree.

The researcher's role is not to *prevent* harm absolutely, since that would bring the clinical and research enterprises, indeed health care itself, to a stop. It is first to value persons, their autonomy, and in consultation with them, to balance benefits and harms in a defensible and evidence-based way (Royal College of Nursing Research Society 2003).

Consequences

This 'risk–benefit' approach could be described as 'consequentialist'. In deciding to conduct a study the research team should carefully assess the risks and benefits that respondents might experience. Where possible, the assessment should be shared with them so that an informed choice can be made. This approach is driven by thought about the outcomes of the study rather than simple adherence to rules or principles, which may be impractical. For example, in respect of any supposed right to privacy, Polit and Hungler (1999) note that:

> *Virtually all research with humans constitutes some type of intrusion into other people's lives.*
>
> (Polit and Hungler 1999)

They go on to suggest that researchers need to minimise this intrusion and to maintain the patient's privacy throughout the study. Clearly they mean that a balance needs to be struck between troubling people for information and making sure that, using the strategies of anonymity and keeping information confidential, their personal lives remain undisclosed in any identifiable way.

In theoretical terms the consequentialist approach has very sound philosophical roots owed mainly to John Stuart Mill (Mill 1972, first published 1910). A 19th Century British intellectual, Mill counted Florence Nightingale among his circle (not that she shared many of his views) and argued forcibly for women's suffrage. He described the 'greatest happiness' principle which:

> *...holds that actions are right in proportion as they tend to promote happiness, wrong as they tend to produce the reverse of happiness. By happiness is intended pleasure, and the absence of pain, by unhappiness, pain and the privation of pleasure.*
>
> (Mill 1972)

Mill's view and use of these terms seems a little dated, and his general principles have been modified greatly in the late 20th Century context by health care philosophers like Harris (1985) and Singer (1993). It may be fair to say that they would now argue that by happiness is meant 'the expression of preferences' and the freedom from pain and discomfort. Perhaps because of the risk of such decisions being made by those in 'authority', in a rare area of consensus these consequentialist philosophers agree with the important 'rights-based' philosopher Immanuel Kant that respect for the *autonomy* of individual persons is the first principle that should be considered in any debate. Johnstone (1994) puts it like this:

> *...people should be free to choose and entitled to act on their preferences provided their decisions and actions do not stand to violate, or impinge upon, the significant moral interests of others.*

(Johnstone 1994)

Autonomy

Autonomy is the ability of an individual to make reasoned decisions about issues that affect them personally. If we respect people, then we must also respect their autonomy, and seek to incorporate their wishes (or preferences) into decisions about their health care and about their participation in health care research (Royal College of Nursing Research Society 2003).

The consequences approach is often said to mean the 'greatest good for the greatest number'. This view is too simplistic, but certainly it means that research that benefits many people in important ways may be said to allow the tolerance of greater discomfort or risk than that which is likely to produce no clear benefit. Such 'calculations', drawing on the views of those likely to be affected if possible, are the proper role of experienced research teams and well-prepared research ethics committees.

In order to evaluate studies from the consequentialist perspective we would usually focus on the outcomes of the study where these can be reasonably known or safely assumed. Depending on the type of study, these might include the relief of suffering for future patients or, less ambitiously, that the study helped to train a new researcher. It is important, however, to attempt an estimate of the inconvenience, discomfort, pain or other risk endured by research participants (including the investigators and other stakeholders). Only then can some evaluation of the relative ethical status of the study be made.

Relational ethics

Researchers commonly find that appealing to traditional rules, codes of conduct and abstract principles helps little in the solution of moral problems faced in day-to-day investigations. It is important to acknowledge that a stronger focus on the processes of research and on 'practical ethics' is owed to the feminist movement. I noted earlier that Gilligan (1982) showed that one of the more popular theories of moral development by Lawrence Kohlberg had failed to examine the moral development of females. Edwards and Mauthner (2002) review contributions to this 'care' or 'relational' perspective noting that there are several inter-related features. They argue that thinking about research dilemmas and problems should include a greater sense of context.

Other ethical theories tend to avoid the social context of the problem on the principle of 'universalisability'. For example, in 'rights-based' thought, if something is wrong then it is *always* wrong. Similarly, from the consequentialist point of view, an action that provides benefit to some participants, should be provided for *all*.

Researchers of any experience, however, will note that even the best-designed quantitative studies can be described as 'messy' with the procedures adopted having to be tailored to local circumstances when the real world is more complex than the proposal could allow. Drawing on the notion of reflexivity feminist researchers have given much greater prominence to personal experience. Reflexivity has been variously defined (Steier 1991) but, in particular, includes the idea of making clear to what extent the researcher, by virtue of their personal experience and selfhood, affects and is affected by the study.

Of special significance to the relational or caring perspective is an acknowledgment that personal relationships affect, and even *should affect* our judgement on moral questions in research. For example, a good deal of educational, practitioner and action research involves a researcher investigating issues of local concern and in which they are directly involved. In contrast to the often spurious 'objective' or 'detached' perspective of traditional ethical approaches, researchers care about the outcome of the study they undertake. In short, they want to make a difference. Reflexivity is a mechanism for making this involvement in the outcome, and the reasons for it, explicit. This explication does not necessarily absolve the researcher from attempting to maintain academic integrity in reporting research outcomes as they were rather than as they would like them to be.

This 'practical ethics' approach (Williams 1991) emphasises the degree to which codes of conduct, protocols, rules and theories are only partially helpful in resolving dilemmas in the research context. Among other criteria by which a feminist perspective can shed light on the important issues, a critical evaluation from this viewpoint should ask what the balance of personal and social power is between those involved (Edwards & Mauthner 2002).

CONCLUSION

To summarise, in health and social care research there are three broad positions from which to view the design and execution of research. Arguably most influential in the form of codes of conduct for research practice is that of human rights. Such codes and statements of rights are useful in that they often have explicit criteria that must be met, and can add a margin of safety for inexperienced researchers. The second or consequential approach is least often admitted to directly, since when not fully understood it can seem to imply that 'anything goes' provided society benefits. When a full appreciation of the importance of individual autonomy and respect for persons is brought into the discussion, it can be seen that this is the pre-eminent model of decision-making in both health care and health and social care research.

Of greater importance recently is a relational or 'care' approach, which has developed in concert with raised consciousness of women's and other oppressed groups' issues. It may be no coincidence that this perspective is popular in the context of qualitative research, where specific research plans are harder to make and where the needs of individuals are said to be of greater importance. Despite this, qualitative research has also been the medium of some quite debatable conduct (Johnson 1992, Johnson 2004).

This has a bearing on the social context in which research is designed, planned, and approved, which is more complex than textbooks or ethical approval forms allow. I have been able only to allude to a few of the issues surrounding the conduct of studies in an ethically defensible way. Issues of occupational socialisation, professional power, social class, gender, race and culture each have a strong influence on the values that we bring to research and those our participants may hold. The idea that 'unethical research' has necessarily been halted by codes of conduct, research ethics committees or approval bodies is false. Despite these, personal and professional integrity and holding key values are central to defensible approaches to research, even when all might not agree equally with the justifications.

REFERENCES

Barbour R (1985) Dealing with the transsituational demands of professional socialisation. Sociological Review 33(3), 495–531.

Becker H, Geer B, Hughes E, Strauss AL (1961) Boys in white: student culture in a medical school, University of Chicago Press, Chicago.

Beecher H (1966) Ethics and clinical research. New England Journal of Medicine 274(24), 1354–1360.

Benjamin M, Curtis J (1981) Ethics in nursing. Oxford University Press, New York.

Cartwright S (1988) The Report of the Cervical Cancer Inquiry. Government Printing Office, Auckland.

Clarke L (1996) Participant observation in a secure unit: care conflict and control. NT Research 1(6), 431–440.

Dew K, Roorda M (2001) Institutional innovation and the handling of health complaints in New Zealand: an assessment. Health Policy 57(1), 27–44.

Department of Health (DH) (2001) The Royal Liverpool Children's Inquiry Report. The Stationery Office, London.

Edwards R, Mauthner M (2002) Ethics and feminist research: theory and practice. In: Mauthner M, Birch M, Jessop J, Miller T (eds) Ethics in qualitative research. Sage, London.

Edwards S (1996) Nursing ethics: a principle–based approach. MacMillan, London.

Field D (1989) Nursing the dying. Tavistock Routledge, London.

Foucault M (1991) Discipline and punish. Penguin, Harmondsworth.

Freidson E (1970) Profession of Medicine. Dodd Mead, New York.

Gilligan C (1982) In a different voice: psychological theory and women's development. Harvard University Press, Cambridge, Mass.

Goffman E (1968) Asylums. Penguin, Harmondsworth.

Gunaratnam Y (2003) Researching 'race' and ethnicity: methods, knowledge and power. Sage, London.

Harris J (1985) The value of life. Routledge and Kegan Paul, London.

Humm C, Lehane M (2005) Time to shout from the rooftops. Nursing Standard 19(47), 32–33.

Humphreys L (1975) The tearoom trade. Aldine, Chicago.

Illich I (1976) Limits to medicine. Marion Boyars, London.

Johnson M (1983) Nurses' values and nurse training: a pilot survey of the values of student nurses. MSc Thesis, Department of Nursing, University of Manchester, Manchester.

Johnson M (1992) A silent conspiracy? some ethical issues of participant observation in nursing research. International Journal of Nursing Studies 29(2), 213–223.

Johnson M (1997) Nursing power and social judgement. Ashgate, Aldershot.

Johnson M (2004) Real world ethics and nursing research. NT Research, now Journal of Research in Nursing 9(4), 251–261.

Johnson M (2005) Notes on the tension between privacy and surveillance in nursing. In: On–Line Journal of Issues in Nursing. Vol.10 No.2, Manuscript 3, Vol. 2005 Kent State University, USA.

Johnstone M (1994) Bioethics: a nursing perspective. WB Saunders, Sydney.

Kramer M (1974) Reality shock: why nurses leave nursing. Mosby, St Louis.

Lacey E (1994) Research utilization in nursing practice: a pilot study. Journal of Advanced Nursing 19(5), 987–995.

Lawler J (1991) Behind the screens: nursing, somology and the problem of the body. Churchill Livingstone, Melbourne.

Lawton J (2000) The dying process: Patients' experiences of palliative care. Routledge, London.

Long T (2004) Excessive Crying in Infancy. Whurr Publishing Ltd, London.

Melia K (1987) Learning and working: the occupational socialisation of student nurses. Tavistock, London.

Mill J S (1972, first published 1910.) Utilitarianism, on liberty and considerations on representative government. J M Dent and Sons Ltd, London.

Moskop JC, Marco CA, Larkin GL, Gelderman JM, Derse AR (2005) From Hippocrates to HIPAA: Privacy and confidentiality in emergency medicine – Part II: Challenges in the emergency department. Annals of Emergency Medicine 45(1), 60–67.

Neville L, Haigh C (2003) A response to Martin Johnson's Editorial "Research ethics and education: a consequentialist view." Nurse Education Today 23(8), 549–553.

Newell R (2002) Research and its relationship to nurse education: Focus and capacity. Nurse Education Today 22(4), 278–284.

Polit D, Hungler B (1999) Nursing Research: Principles and Methods. Lippincott, Philadelphia.

Psathas G (1968) The fate of idealism in nursing school. Journal of Health and Social Behaviour 9, 52–64.

Rosenhan D (1973) On being sane in insane places. Science 179, 250–258.

Singer P (1993) Practical ethics. Cambridge University Press, Cambridge.

Steier F (1991) Research and reflexivity. Sage, London.

The Royal College of Nursing Research Society (2003) Nurses and research ethics. Nurse Researcher 11(1), 7–21.

The Victoria Climbié Inquiry (2003) Report of an inquiry by Lord Laming presented to Parliament by the Secretary of State for Health and the Secretary of State for the Home Department by Command of Her Majesty. The Stationery Office, London.

Walsh K, Kowanko I (2002) Nurses' and patients' perceptions of dignity. International Journal of Nursing Practice 8, 143–151.

Williams A (1991) Practical ethics: interpretive processes in an ethnography of nursing. In: Aldridge J, Griffiths V, Williams A (eds) Rethinking: Feminist research processes reconsidered, vol. 34 Feminist Praxis: Studies in Sexual Politics, Manchester.

WMA (2005) World medical association declaration of Helsinki. Vol. 2005 The World Medical Association, Ferney–Voltaire.

Woolhead G, Calnan M, Dieppe P, Tadd W (2004) Dignity in older age: what do older people in the United Kingdom think? Age and Ageing 33(2), 165–170.

4

What are the ethical issues in research?

Tony Long

The previous chapter established the basis for concern about the welfare of research participants and subjects and the foundation for the need to uphold their rights and respect their decisions. This chapter and the next turn to the issues that arise in research with human participants and how these may be addressed satisfactorily. In particular, the notion of harm or risk to the participant is crucial here. Issues in three main areas should be borne in mind by the researcher:

1. Concerns regarding coercion, deception, information, and voluntary participation in research (consent)
2. Factors relating to the divulging of personal information (confidentiality)
3. Matters pertaining to particular groups of individuals whose characteristics imply additional vulnerability or the need for additional effort to ensure appropriate treatment.

RISKS TO PARTICIPANTS IN RESEARCH

Risks, or the potential for harm, may present in many forms for research participants. For some, the risk of physical harm is significant. For example, the testing of exercise tolerance in heart disease must be carefully monitored in order to prevent adverse events. While the results are expected to be life-enhancing or even life-saving, experimental surgery or other medical treatment may bear the risk of causing disfigurement, lasting disability, or even death. Such high stakes may be acceptable to the patient as research subject, but the risk remains to be taken into account.

Unanticipated side-effects can exert a catastrophic impact on people's lives. A classic example of this was the introduction of the drug Thalidomide in the late 1950s. Animal tests had produced results that suggested that there were no harmful side-effects.

Tests on healthy human volunteers had also shown no observable negative effects. It was only after the drug had been administered to women in the first trimester of pregnancy that the terrible teratogenic effects were discovered. This served as a painful reminder that only tests on the target population can show the true effect, and the possibility of unforeseen side-effects remains an issue for researchers and participants to consider carefully. Thalidomide is now in use again as an effective agent in the treatment of skin lesions in leprosy, and it may have potential to inhibit the growth of HIV infection by suppressing a natural substance known as tumour necrosis factor (TNF).

A less severe, though far more common, side-effect is that of research participants suffering discomfort, fatigue or boredom. Experiments in sleeping patterns and disruption of sleep are a prime example of this. In some sleep experiments the subject is woken up every time they enter rapid eye movement (REM) sleep (the dream state) leading to them becoming increasingly impatient and uncomfortable over time. Other experiments require the wearing of electrodes on the head, sensors to observe eye movement, a tight-fitting vest to monitor respiratory effort in the chest and diaphragm (a respiratory inductance plethysmograph vest for the more technical mind), or other sensors to monitor body movement (Fig. 4.1).

Emotional distress is another possible risk for participants in research studies. It takes little imagination to visualise the possibilities. Interviewing victims of social disadvantage, personal tragedy, family strife and so on clearly seeks to elicit data that has huge potential to provoke distress, grief and all manner of emotional reaction. Without denying this, it might be recognised, however, that such distress is a natural part of life in general. It is, perhaps, a matter of degree. Some degree of upset may be acceptable (a normal part of day-to-day life) while more intense distress requires more justification. Questions that rouse wistful memories or a tearful response may be seen in a different light to data collection that provokes the need for professional therapeutic intervention. Nevertheless, if progress is to be made through research in some areas of health and social care then a degree of minor (or even more serious) emotional distress may be both allowable and necessary. In the next chapter this will be explained more fully as the activity of risk–benefit analysis.

Occasionally, the risk to participants may be the loss of privacy. This may take the form of having to discuss personal habits, beliefs or experiences or it may involve photographic or videotape

Fig 4.1 US Senator John H Glenn Jr taking part in sleep experiments on board Space Shuttle STS-95 (Reproduced by permission of NASA)

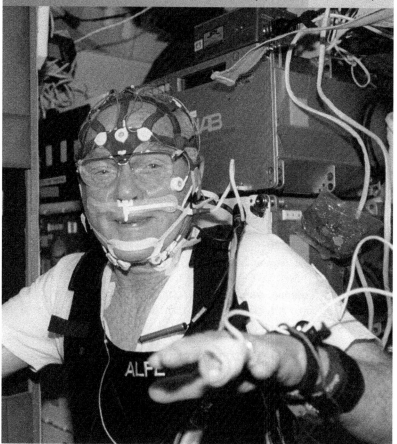

recording of the body; perhaps in research into deformity, abnormal gait, or treatment of skin lesions. However much the research team may be trusted, the recording and storage of such data can cause concern, while inadvertent or insensitive presentation of images as part of the dissemination of findings can cause far more distress. There is the danger, too, of sensitive information being unintentionally divulged (perhaps to an employer or government agency) to the detriment of the subject's employment or financial interests. Sometimes, the risk of loss of privacy is presented by other research participants. This is the case with focus-group interviews. While it is usual to agree ground rules at the beginning of the process and to remind participants of the need for confidentiality at the closure of the interview, the maintenance of this cannot be guaranteed.

Research participants can be surprised (and dismayed) at the amount of their time that may be taken up in a study. Travel, waiting, undertaking tests, completing questionnaires and so on, can exert a cumulative effect, sometimes involving considerable financial cost, too. Classically, market research may draw the subject in gradually: 'Do you have just two minutes to complete a brief questionnaire?' (2 minutes later). 'Thanks for that. May I just check a few details now?' (5 minutes later). 'That's really helpful. I've almost finished. You've been really good. Would you just look at these pictures to finish off and tell me your impressions of them?' (15 minutes later...). Of course, this is a parody only of less reputable market research, but the format will be recognised by many.

There are, then, many potential harms that can befall the research participant however well informed and willing they may be, and these need to be considered carefully by the researcher when designing the study. For the most part these issues fall broadly into three areas of concern, which will be considered in more detail now.

VOLUNTARY PARTICIPATION IN RESEARCH

Showing respect for individuals and groups and upholding their rights includes allowing them to make decisions for themselves about issues that impact on them. Accordingly, it is generally held that undertaking research on or with individuals normally should be pursued only with their full knowledge and consent. In this sense consent means that the individual has access to adequate information about the proposed study and their involvement in it, that they are able to make a reasoned decision as to whether or not to participate, and that they are not under undue pressure to be involved. These three elements are all essential for the participant's consent to be valid.

Competence

Competence relates to the ability of an individual to process information about an issue or topic, to reason about the relevant factors and their own preferences or values, and to express their consequent judgement or decision (even if this be foolish, capricious or ill-advised). Importantly, as will be seen shortly, competence is best viewed not as an all-or-nothing concept, but as a variable quality relative to the circumstances of the case and the nature of the associated risk of harm. For the researcher the task is to gauge the seriousness of the decision to be made and the degree of competence required on the part of the individual for consent to be considered valid.

Children are often too readily dismissed as being too immature to be competent. Even at a very early age, however, children show the ability to discriminate between options and to express preferences as to what they should do or what others should be allowed to do with or to them. At this end of the lifespan it is wiser to consider competence as an incremental ability that develops as the child grows older, linked through a period of shared decision-making to a phased reduction in the parental role to make decisions on behalf of the child.

Similarly, confusion in older people may promote premature dismissal of their ability to make rational decisions. Commonplace as confusion may be, it is equally common for confusion to be patchy rather than complete, and many older people who display confusion in some aspects of their lives are perfectly capable of thinking clearly about complex issues in other aspects. They may, indeed, have the advantage of additional years of experience and reflection on which to base a reasoned decision.

Competence may be temporarily diminished as in the case of someone who has become suddenly and seriously ill; mentally or physically. In such cases competence may be expected to return with recovery and decisions must be made about whether or not participation can be delayed until this point. Once again, however, the misfortune of mental illness does not automatically preclude the ability to make reasoned decisions and, with skilled help, it is usually possible to determine the likelihood of valid consent in individual cases. For some people competence ceases with no possibility of return (perhaps in catastrophic brain injury or even death), and in these circumstances alternative approaches to protecting the welfare of participants are required.

On occasion a study may be completed without any reference to the participants, either in the form of providing information or in gaining consent. Examples of this include the on-going Unlinked Anonymous Prevalence Monitoring Programme (UAPMP) designed to establish the distribution of undiagnosed infection (and particularly HIV) in the adult population of the UK (Health Protection Agency 2005). The study began in 1990 and by 2005 had analysed almost eight million samples of human tissue, largely from pregnant women and attenders at genito-urinary medicine clinics. In cases such as this anonymity is protected through measures to remove any link between the sample and the identity of the donor, and the focus is upon populations rather than individuals.

Information

Decisions in every aspect of life are generally reliant on the acquisition of adequate information, whether buying a new car, choosing a school for children, or selecting food for a healthy diet. Similarly, decisions about participating in research should be based on reasoning about adequate, truthful information. Two factors present in this regard: the content of the information and the effectiveness of its presentation.

Before agreeing to participate in a research study it should be clear what this participation might entail. Completing a questionnaire may appear an innocuous demand until it becomes clear that doing so requires the divulging of highly personal information; agreeing to be videotaped walking along a marked path may seem reasonable until it is established that this must be done naked. Attending for additional clinic visits to have extra blood tests may feel more onerous when it is discovered that the plan is for this to continue for 5 years. Informed participation, then, involves being aware of precisely what demands will be placed on a recruit and what the boundaries may be of participation. The information should include details of major risks, other treatment options (apart from those offered to participants) and any elements that are simply not known for certain.

Information, however accurate, is of little use if it cannot be received or understood, and the presentation of information is a vital aspect of ensuring informed choices. Issues of readability of printed information are important; for adults as well as for children. It is easy for academics and professionals to produce technical information speckled with jargon and written in a tortuous academic style that confuses the reader and masks important details. Language can also be a problem for those whose first language is not English. Even the carefully constructed universal proforma prescribed by the Central Office for Research Ethics Committees (COREC)[1] can appear as an oppressive instrument in some circumstances, particularly when the presentation is alien to the experience of the recruit. Alternative forms of communication

---

[1] http://www.corec.org.uk

are more appropriate for some, especially young children and many people with a disability (perhaps blindness). Pictorial presentation, aural materials and less formal interactive approaches may be more useful. It is essential that the circumstances of the proposed participants drive the mode of presenting information.

Coercion

Clearly, even if adequate and truthful information has been provided for a competent individual to make an informed choice, coercion in the form of moral force, power differential or threat of retribution, could easily prevent the free choice of options. Such external pressure can be brought to bear unwittingly by researchers, notably in the choice of colleagues or students as research participants, but also through excessive zeal in recruitment.

The use of students, particularly the researcher's own students or those from the same institution where the researcher may exert some influence (such as marking assessed work), provokes difficulties due to the power differential between lecturer and student (see Chapter 3). Similar problems accrue when subordinate staff members are recruited for a research study. Concern about retribution consequent upon refusing to participate, eagerness to remain on good terms with a superior, or perceptions of a lack of legitimate free choice, may persuade an individual to participate on a less than willing basis. The situation of patients or service users invited to participate in research conducted or supported by health professionals who are responsible for medical management or other health intervention is equally fraught with the potential for unintended coercion. Patients may be especially anxious to receive the most effective treatment option (perhaps, on occasion, the only treatment option), and any price may seem worth paying. In a clear-cut case where the alternative option to experimental treatment is death, then, outrageous side-effects apart, the willingness of a patient to participate may be quite understandable. Yet such cases are not the norm, and other treatment options are more usually available. Sometimes the outcomes from experimental treatments (and the associated risk of harm) are completely unpredictable, and more concern will be shown in these circumstances that undue pressure is not allowed to influence the potential participant's decision.

Misguided notions of priorities (the need to get the research completed in order to offer improvement to many, for example) may also allow undue influence to be exerted on the potential recruit's decision-making. This may be exacerbated by the health professional's training to persuade individuals and groups to adopt behaviours that enhance health and reduce health risks. The distinctions between persuasion and coercion can become blurred, particularly when people appear determined to make apparently unwise choices. Acting in someone's overt best interest may conflict with respecting their right to free choice.

Consent

Continued consent Some research projects address changes in data over long periods of time; often years. In such cases it is important that consent gained at the beginning of the study remains valid later on. While there is no universal rule for this, it is common to consider reviewing the on-going nature of consent periodically. The Royal College of Nursing, for example, recommends review every 6 months (Royal College of Nursing 2005). Regular review may be inappropriate (perhaps when periods of participation are not regular) and in this case it may be more useful to check on the participant's continued willingness to be involved at each period of data collection, rather than at regular intervals.

Implied consent It is possible for individuals to indicate consent by their actions rather than by verbal affirmation. As well as the classic series of codes such as blinking once for 'Yes' and twice for 'No' portrayed in films, it may be that a patient is clearly in agreement to a proposed action because they act in response to the request. They may offer their arm for a blood test to be taken, or they may indicate that a relative should provide information and confirm this with a nod, for example. This may well constitute valid consent, though the researcher should be careful to ensure that it is expressed on an informed basis and not simply compliance with perceived medical treatment.

Assumed consent and delayed consent It may not always be possible to foresee that an individual will become a candidate for recruitment to a study. A study, for example, into nurses' verbal intervention with partially conscious, seriously injured casualties in an accident and emergency department could not begin if the normal processes of providing information to a competent participant had to be completed first. In this instance, provided that the risk to the participant is minimal and the likely benefit from the research is significant (to be addressed more fully below) the study may begin. This would be under the assumption that a reasonable patient would probably not object and with the intention to complete the normal requirements for recruitment at the earliest time possible. If at that time the patient objected, then the data would have to be destroyed.

In other situations there may be the possibility of offering general information to a wider population that may be at variable risk of meeting the requirements for entry to a study. An example of this might be the providing of 'routine' information to all patients admitted to a hospital that a study is being conducted into physiological responses during cardiac arrest, and that if individuals wish to decline being included 'in the very unlikely event of their being found to need resuscitation', they need only tell one of the staff. This is somewhat better than the previous scenario, but without the proximity of the event and the belief that this may be a real possibility for the individual it might be questioned whether or not individuals had really considered the matter as seriously as might be desired. Yet there is a line to draw between promoting an informed decision and offering so much information as to provoke unnecessary distress and undue anxiety in patients.

False consent There are circumstances in which providing full and accurate information about the study would exert such impacts on the participants' behaviour as to negate the value of the research altogether (see, for example, Stockwell 1972, 1984). In such circumstances, the recruit may be offered information that is incomplete or misleading before the study and informed of the truth only after participation. Clearly, this amounts to deception and firm justification is needed, particularly relating to the strength of likely benefits compared with the liberty of the deception, and to the unavailability of any other means of undertaking the study.

Evidence of consent The emergence of COREC and standardised documentation for ethical approval throughout the UK has led to common principles for the formulation of the consent form for use in research studies. This is not compulsory, but in practice convincing reasons must be given for the use of alternatives. What is of interest is what is thought to be evidenced by the completion of this form. The form centres on declarations by the recruit that the researcher has undertaken certain functions and that they (the participant) agree to be recruited to the study. It clearly offers something to the researcher (apparent proof of having acted properly), but what it fails to do is to offer guarantees to the participant. There is no indicator of what will happen should things go wrong, for example. In fact, it represents no guarantee at all that recruitment was subject to an informed and voluntary decision on the part of the respondent, yet much is believed to rest upon the completion and storing of these consent forms.

In clinical practice it is common for patients to be completely unable to explain the reasons that necessitated the surgery evidenced by healed scars on the abdomen. Yet the surgery would not have been performed without a signed consent form. This is not a suggestion that surgical teams do not try hard to provide essential information to patients or that the patients sign consent forms reluctantly: quite the opposite. The point is that many patients will sign without really understanding the anatomical or physiological problem at issue, the nature of the proposed surgery or the risks involved. If they do that in the obviously dangerous case of major surgery, it is no surprise that they do it in the case of research, too.

Of course, being required to obtain signed consent forms may make it more difficult for an unscrupulous researcher to act improperly, but it would represent a step forward if a more consumer-orientated perspective were adopted. In most other undertakings (such as the purchase of goods, for example) in which protection of the consumer is the aim, it is the selling organisation (in this example, corresponding to the researcher) that provides the guarantees. Evidence is expected from the vendor that certain guarantees are in place to redress any harm or loss resulting from the sale. This may be expected by a research ethics committee before approval is granted, but the signing of a consent form does not represent this guarantee. However, as with a purchase of goods or services, at least it is expected that the consumer (research participant) will retain a signed copy of the consent form. The important issue is that researchers and those governing access to patients and other vulnerable research participants recognise the limitations of consent forms as guarantees of ethical conduct and evidence of valid consent.

CONFIDENTIALITY

Another aspect of respecting people's autonomous rights that impacts on research is the protection of the identity of participants (where appropriate and desirable). Data that may be sensitive in this way include, among many other elements, personal information, biographical details, medical history and particulars about relationships. Each of these may be essential to the study in question, but on the whole such information should be used only to facilitate data analysis and to promote more meaningful results and recommendations. Rarely would this sort of information be divulged beyond the research team, and serious efforts must be made to prevent accidental disclosure to third parties. When respondents allow researchers to breach their normal privacy and offer access to personal information that may be damaging or embarrassing if released, for example, to the public, employers, or colleagues, then this implies a contract with the researcher to respect the nature of the information and to guard its confidential nature responsibly.

It would be a mistake to think that only details held on paper constitute any threat to confidentiality. Information may be stored in a variety of electronic formats, while the nature of data is becoming noticeably more varied. Respondents may express themselves in drama, painting or sculpture, and data are often collected on videotape, photographs and oral recordings. Each of these presents particular problems for the researcher in providing secure storage, and some modes of data collection pose additional threats to security, especially on-line data collection through the Internet (see Chapter 10).

As in professional life generally, there are circumstances in which the maintenance of confidentiality may be morally (and legally) indefensible, and controlled disclosure to an appropriate authority can be the right course of action. The most important of these is the discovery by the researcher of a serious threat to the respondent or a third party that may be realised if no action is taken. Confidentiality cannot, then, be absolutely guaranteed, but such events are thankfully rare.

ISSUES RELATING TO PARTICULAR GROUPS OF PARTICIPANTS

Some groups of people are, by their nature, often more vulnerable than most to exploitation through research. Children, by virtue of their still-developing competence, and their parents, because of anxiety for their child's wellbeing, clearly require particular attention when researchers seek to include them in a study. It will be seen that varied techniques of information-giving and dialogue are often needed to engage children fully in the decision-making process. Even very young primary school children can hold well-informed views on issues that relate to them once information has been provided in appropriate ways, and proper efforts on the researcher's part can lead to effective expressing of their wishes and values. It is accepted that when children are unable to play a full part in deciding whether or not to participate in research then their parents are normally in the best position and hold the best motivation to decide on their behalf. There are, of course, exceptions to this rule, but parental rights and responsibilities should not be over-ruled too readily. For children in the care of social services, and when an appropriate legal guardian is responsible for decision-making on the child's behalf, it is good practice to keep parents informed of decisions. In either case, when an adult makes decisions for a child in this way the researcher should be sure, at least, that the child does not object to participation.

In England and Wales (and separately in Scotland) guidance for appropriate behaviour in research with children is offered through the law on consent to medical treatment, with additional guidance from the Department of Health, the Medical Research Council and other bodies (Medical Research Council 2004, Department of Health 2001). Application to research with children is not explicit, but in the absence of any specific legislation it is reasonable to assume that the law on medical treatment also applies to medical research. The law in England is based both on statute and on a number of cases. The Family Law Reform Act (1969) laid the basis that has stood the test of time that minors over 16 years may give consent to treatment independently (i.e. without parental consent), but individuals must be 18 years or more to refuse treatment that is considered necessary or advisable by doctor. This did not invalidate parental consent whatever the age of the child. This may seem confusing, but the effect was that children could agree for themselves with what is assumed to be good advice, but not go against (assumed) sound medical advice. Parental consent was always required for a child of less than 16 years.

The latter aspect was revised as a result of the Gillick case (Gillick v West Norfolk and Wisbech AHA 1984, 1985). Mrs Gillick sought a legal declaration that advice and treatment of a minor must not be allowed without parental consent or knowledge. (The specific case related to contraceptive treatment and advice.) She lost her case in the High Court on the grounds that the doctor's action would be no more legal if she had agreed to it, but in the Court of Appeal (1985) she won. The judgement was that the parent's rights extended beyond deciding about treatment for a minor to include medical advice. However, in a landmark decision in the House of Lords the case was finally lost. The rationale was that the welfare of the child must be paramount.

This appeared to resolve the matter: if the child was of sufficient understanding to make a decision for themselves and refused to allow their parent to be consulted then they could offer (or refuse) consent independently.

If and when the child achieves a sufficient understanding and intelligence to enable him to understand fully what is proposed he is treated as having the capacity to give a valid consent to medical treatment.

Gillick v West Norfolk and Wisbech Area Health Authority
[1986] AC 112

Two cases since then have undercut the Gillick decision. In Re R (1991) an adolescent girl in a psychiatric unit was denied the right to act as a 'Gillick competent' minor and her parent was allowed to insist on medical treatment. In Re W (1992), W was 16 years old and refused treatment. The judgement was, however, that parental rights were not terminated by the decision of a competent minor. This clearly was a direct refutation of the Gillick principle, and other cases have followed in a similar vein such that the notion of the Gillick competent child has become seriously undermined.

In England, Wales and Northern Ireland the Children Act 1989 and the Children Act (Northern Ireland) Order 1995 provide for parental rights and responsibilities with regard to their children, including the right (and responsibility) to make decisions on behalf of incompetent children in cases of medical treatment. Again, the principle of the child's welfare being paramount is upheld, and the law allows for a parent to over-rule their competent child's refusal of treatment likely to be beneficial.

In Scotland, the Age of Legal Capacity (Scotland) Act 1991 addresses the right of young people under 16 years of age to consent to medical treatment, provided they are capable of understanding the nature and possible consequences of the procedure or treatment. Additionally, the Children (Scotland) Act 1995 provides guidance in the case of children of less than 16 years of age who are not competent. A further statute – the Adults with Incapacity (Scotland) Act 2000 – addresses the approach to young people of 16 and 17 years who are incompetent to give consent.

The Medical Research Council offers clear guidance on involving children in research (Medical Research Council 2004). The key principles are reproduced in Box 4.1. The MRC allows for only a negligible risk of harm to children if participating in non-therapeutic research, and demands that possible risks must be outweighed by likely benefits in therapeutic research with children.

Other groups may cause additional concern as research subjects or participants. Research with pregnant women involves recognition of the women's rights as individuals, but concern will also be felt for the wellbeing of the foetus. Research on or with older people who are unable to give consent should be avoided if the study could be carried out equally well with competent older adults. If the nature of the research prevents this (for example,

---

Box 4.1 Summary of key ethical principles relating to research involving children (MRC 2004)

- Research should include children only where the relevant knowledge cannot be obtained by research in adults.
- The purpose of the research is to obtain knowledge relevant to the health, wellbeing or health-care needs of children.
- Researchers can involve competent children only if they have obtained their informed consent beforehand.
- A child's refusal to participate or continue in research should always be respected.
- If a child becomes upset by a procedure researchers must accept this as a valid refusal.
- Researchers should involve parents/guardians in the decision to participate wherever possible, and in all cases where the child is not yet competent. (There may be exceptional circumstances to this.)
- Researchers should attempt to avoid any pressures that might lead the child to volunteer for research or that might lead parents to volunteer their children in the expectation of direct benefit (whether therapeutic or financial).
- Research involves partnership with the child and/or family who should be kept informed and consent to separate stages of the project. Obtaining consent is a continuing process rather than a one-off occurrence. Children and their families are likely to appreciate some recognition of their role in this partnership, such as a certificate of participation.
- Researchers must take account of the cumulative medical, emotional, social and psychological consequences of the child being involved in research. Children with certain conditions may be exposed to a sequence of research projects. It is advisable to consider the risks of a particular research procedure in the context of the child's overall involvement in projects by different researchers.

responses to a drug for a specific, disabling condition), then the study should be carried out only if the individual stands to benefit, or at least will not be harmed while others will benefit. The same principles apply to research with people with disability and those with mental illness. Consistency can be seen, then, in the approach to a range of vulnerable people. The first aim should be to foster informed decisions by the individuals to whatever extent this is possible, and then to place the welfare of the participant first. If justification is found to include subjects who are not completely competent, then continuation of the study should be dependent upon the individual at least not objecting to participation.

In all such instances a balanced approach is required. The advancement of treatment and care for vulnerable groups, just as for any other group, is dependent upon sound research. Preventing research with such groups on the basis of the difficulty of gaining valid consent risks the imposition of a situation of double jeopardy in which those already at disadvantage are further disadvantaged because of their existing difficulty. If the medical or social condition of individuals could be enhanced through research, then denying them access to this (by preventing the conduct of responsible research) compounds their misfortune. A similar effect, though for a rather different reason, applies to the frequent exclusion of people from research studies because of their inability alternatively to speak, hear, read or write English. Despite the additional difficulties of providing appropriate information and then conducting the study, researchers risk denying another potentially vulnerable group the benefits of the results of research if they are too readily excluded.

Sound arguments are forwarded by Gelling for research with patients in persistent vegetative state: a group that has been chronically under-researched by neuroscientists because complex ethical questions and logistical dilemmas are raised by such research (Gelling 2004). Gelling demonstrates that not only is it possible to undertake such research, but that it is essential to do so in order that greater numbers of patients and their families will benefit.

CONCLUSION

The risks to participants in research studies arise in many forms and to varying degrees of significance. Many can be foreseen, but some outcomes will always be unpredictable. In addition to the effects of the research on the participant, issues of competence to decide about participation, the suitability of information provided, protection of confidential information and problems relating to specific groups of participants must all be understood by the researcher. A thoughtful, balanced perspective on each individual case is required, and this depends upon due recognition of the risks involved and the needs of those whose participation is sought.

REFERENCES

Department of Health (2001) Consent - what you have a right to expect. A guide for children and young people. DH, London.

Gelling L (2004) Researching patients in the vegetative state: difficulties of studying this patient group. NT Research 9(1), 7–17.

Health Protection Agency (2005) The Unlinked Anonymous Prevalence Monitoring Programme. HPA, London.

Medical Research Council (2004) Medical research involving children. MRC, London.

Royal College of Nursing (2005) Informed consent in health and social care research: RCN guidance for nurses. RCN, London.

Stockwell F (1972, 1984) The unpopular patient. Croom Helm, London.

LEGAL REFERENCES

Gillick v West Norfolk and Wisbech AHA [1986] AC 112, [1985] 3 WLR 830, [1985] 3 All ER 402, HL

Age of Legal Capacity (Scotland) Act 1991

Children Act 1989

Children Act (Northern Ireland) Order 1995

Children (Scotland) Act 1995

Adults with Incapacity (Scotland) Act 2000

Family Law Reform Act 1969

Re R (a minor) (wardship: medical treatment) [1991] 7 BMLR 147

Re W (a minor) (medical treatment) [1992] 4 All ER 627

5

How are these ethical issues to be resolved?

Tony Long

The most important device for addressing the ethical issues discussed in Chapter 4 is the notion of risk–benefit analysis. This requires the researcher to identify the possible risks to individuals of involvement in the study and to weigh these against the potential benefit to the individual of participating. In general terms, the potential harms should be outweighed by the potential benefits or additional, particularly convincing justification is needed. Furthermore, for each identified risk of harm the researcher should plan specific, relevant measures to eliminate the risk, to minimise the impact of the risk should it be realised, or to cope with (or compensate for) any harm that eventually accrues to the participant.

POTENTIAL BENEFITS FROM PARTICIPATION IN RESEARCH

The more common risks, associated with being a research participant, have been outlined in the previous chapter. Risk–benefit analysis requires balancing of these against potential benefits, of which there may be many, few, or even none at all. Unfortunately, such balancing relies upon an unscientific process in which risks and potential benefits cannot usually actually be measured. Instead, subjective judgement is required, and because of this there is always an element of uncertainty about the resulting decision.

For some, access to an otherwise unavailable treatment may represent adequate recompense for the inconvenience or even danger of participation. This has been the case with some new treatments for AIDS, for example. With an otherwise gloomy prognosis, any chance of effective treatment can seem inviting. There is often an instinctive negative public (and sometimes professional) reaction to experimental treatment. This may be justified sometimes, but clear thinking is needed before rushing into a gut-based judgement. It is important to distinguish between experimental treatment when a reasonably satisfactory alternative exists (that is, when the risk is high and the alternative is reasonably positive) and when no alternative exists; other than death. In the latter case, and with only one proviso, the experimental treatment offers at least an equal possibility to the existing option and possibly a significantly better outcome. The patient stands only to gain or at least to be no worse off. The proviso, of course, is that the nature (including side-effects) of the treatment could involve so much suffering or discomfort as to be considered possibly worse than death. The decision about whether or not the potential benefit is worth the risk must lie ultimately with the patient.

Anyone who suffers from chronic back pain will know how quickly interest and sympathy run out in third parties. Participating in a research study can offer such a sufferer the benefit of discussing their history, complaints, problems and feelings with someone who desperately wants to listen; a rare enough phenomenon in many instances. This attention can in itself be therapeutic, both to the sufferer and their carer, as well as to others with the same condition through the results of the study.

Increased knowledge of their own medical condition, or insight into their social circumstances or behaviour could be a real benefit to some people. The popularity of television programmes in which an expert solves problems for individuals relating to financial difficulties, obesity, smoking habits or relationship problems seems to bear witness to the value of individual attention in such matters. The individual attention of an expert in the field with a serious interest in their particular case could be especially inviting for many. The respectful attention of the researcher, together with relevant explanations and expressions of the value of the participant's contribution may serve to enhance their self-esteem, restoring feelings of self-worth and the social acceptability of their personal circumstances.

Sadly, participating in research may offer a welcome break from the monotony and routine of daily life, particularly so if an individual's existence is limited by immobility (perhaps being housebound by arthritis), restricted by authority (an issue for some young people in child and family psychiatric units some of the time), or simply restrained by financial limitations. The potential for exploitation may be particularly acute in such circumstances, but once again, only the participant is able to make a truly valid judgement of the relative merits of risks and benefits.

The altruistic satisfaction of having helped others (in a similar situation or not) should not be underestimated. In a society where blood donation is undertaken without financial reward, and where voluntary work is so common it may not be surprising that so many people are prepared to act as research subjects simply in order to make a contribution to society or those in less advantageous circumstances.

The issue of payment for such service is a recurring problem. Of course, much research is undertaken by paying subjects for their time and inconvenience. Commercial radio stations frequently broadcast advertisements for volunteers to act as research subjects in this manner. The main concern in this area is that those already suffering the greatest disadvantage may be the ones most easily targeted, and relatively small payment may be required to secure participation in research with significant risk of harm. Certainly, many students supplement their meagre incomes in this manner. Payment for children's participation as research subjects is especially difficult to manage. Helpful guidance is offered by (INVOLVE 2004).

Predicting the benefits of a particular study can be difficult even with the most rigorous of experiments. In qualitative research with less foreseeable outcomes this estimation can be even harder to make. For this reason approval committees and other gate-keepers sometimes find it difficult to approve such studies. However, the more that such studies are undertaken the greater the likelihood that some may be very beneficial, and few would doubt the influence and importance of works of this kind by Barney Glaser and Anselm Strauss (Glaser & Strauss 1965), which drew attention to the way the dying were treated; by Felicity Stockwell (Stockwell 1972, 1984) who explored the inappropriate labelling of patients; and, more recently, by Julia Lawton (Lawton 2000) who shows clearly how grim the process of dying, even in a hospice, can actually be.

ENSURING EFFECTIVE CONSENT TO PARTICIPATE

A number of routine measures that are usually a matter simply of good practice and that have become commonly accepted and expected should be firmly within the researcher's repertoire of skills. For less generic risks and for unforeseen circumstances a more active engagement with the process of risk–benefit analysis is needed. Of the routine measures, gaining valid consent from participants is the first and most important.

Providing information

The most common medium for the provision of information is printed sheets. These commonly now use the question and answer format recommended by the Central Office for Research Ethics Committees (COREC) (see Box 5.1). The general purpose of this is to make the information more accessible to potential participants and to reduce ambiguity in the content. Researchers must always bear in mind that individuals' ability to read and understand information may be limited by a number of factors, including limited literacy, problems with English as a foreign language, and problems with vision. Limited knowledge of medical, anatomical and research terminology often compounds this.

A series of guidance booklets is also available from CERES, including *Spreading the word on research - or - patient information: how can we get it better?* (Consumers for Ethics in Research 1994). As well as practical advice this publication offers examples of

---

Box 5.1 The COREC formula for information sheets

The following questions or topics should be addressed. COREC provides detailed advice for some of these sections:
Study title
Invitation paragraph
What is the purpose of the study?
Why have I been chosen?
Do I have to take part?
What will happen to me if I take part?
What do I have to do?
What is the drug or procedure that is being tested? (If appropriate)
What are the alternatives for diagnosis or treatment?
What are the side-effects of any treatment received when taking part?
What are the possible disadvantages and risks of taking part?
What are the possible benefits of taking part?
What if new information becomes available?
What happens when the research study stops?
What if something goes wrong?
Will my taking part in this study be kept confidential?
What will happen to the results of the research study?
Who is organising and funding the research?
Who has reviewed the study?

Contact for further information
http://www.corec.org.uk/applicants/help/docs/Guidance_on_Patient_Information_Sheets_and_Consent_Forms.doc (Correct at 12.03.06)

hopelessly complex information provided to potential research participants together with much simpler alternative means of expressing the same information. It notes, too, that there is a danger of appearing to be patronising, crude or irritating by over-simplifying information (see Box 5.2).

Readability formulae

One of the more common problems with printed information provided for research participants is that it is written in a format and using terminology that requires too high a level of reading ability for some participants. Fortunately, a number of tested devices are available to assist researchers in avoiding this fault. Some word-processing packages (such as MS Word™ for Windows XP™) feature the ability within the spelling and

---

Box 5.2 What to include in information leaflets – guidance from Consumers for Ethics in Research (CERES)

Advice from CERES is formulated less as a template for the final document and more as a series of issues for the researcher to consider in composing the information sheet.

- Who is this for? What might they want to know? How can I tell them? What do I want to tell them?
- The name of the project.
- The problem or question to be addressed.
- The request.
- The hoped-for benefits (Direct or indirect benefit? Uncertainty – benefits are not certain, just hoped for).
- What the request involves – research practice (timing, data collection, confidentiality, risk, harm, cost, indemnity, approval from a research ethics committee).
- What the research involves – research method (treatment v placebo group, data collection method).
- Contact details.
- Any other questions (What new question is being addressed? Who is funding the project? What happens if my treatment emerges as being less effective than another? Will there be any follow-up? Will I be told the research results?).
- Making a decision (Do I have to say yes? Do I have to decide at once? How might the research help me?).

CERES (1994) Spreading the word on research – or – patient information: how can we get it better?

grammar checking tool to calculate readability, but standard tests of readability based on sentence length and other criteria are more often used. An example of one of these is provided in Box 5.3.

Participants for whom English language is a problem

Those for whom speaking, reading, or writing English is problematic have often been excluded from research because of the difficulty in providing adequate information for them and the work involved in preparing additional versions of data-collection instruments. The latter involves financial cost and time, and is too often avoided by researchers. Sadly, excluding this group from involvement in research also denies them the opportunity to have their specific issues, needs and concerns addressed. The results of research studies undertaken with only those whose first language is English may simply not be applicable to (for example) minority ethnic groups.

The reverse of this problem of denying sub-groups the opportunity to benefit from research can be that some individual or groups are persuaded to participate in research studies without understanding essential elements of the study or the risks to themselves. Furthermore, language is not the only issue of concern in such circumstances. Religious and cultural factors will often be significant, too.

Translation of information into other languages is a skilled occupation and, if undertaken without adequate knowledge of cultural and gender issues, can be little short of disastrous. CERES offers a helpful technique to check on the effectiveness and accuracy of translated material; having one individual translate from English into the second language, then having a second individual translate the new version back into English (Consumers for Ethics in Research 2002). The result of this exercise can be stunning.

Information for children

Some children will be able to cope with the normal information sheet, particularly if helped by their parents. Younger children who are not able to do so still require information to enable them to make an informed decision, even though this is likely to be supplementary to parental information and decision-making. An example of an information sheet for children is displayed in Figure 5.1, while an example of an information sheet for parents is offered in Figure 5.2.

Box 5.3 Example of a readability test: The Fog Index

The **Gunning Fog Index** is a readability test designed to show how easy or difficult a text is to read. It uses the following algorithm:

1. Calculate the average number of words used per sentence. This is usually done on a sample of the text (15–20 lines).
   (Number of words divided by the number of sentences)
2. Calculate the percentage of 'difficult' words in the text. A difficult word is one which is three syllables or more long, but excluding proper nouns such as the name of a city (for example, 'Manchester'), simple words joined together into a larger one (for example, 'highlighted'), and words that are three syllables only because of suffixes (–ing, –ed).
   (Difficult words X 100, divided by total number of words)
3. Add these figures together, then multiply by 0.4.
   (Average words per sentence + percentage of difficult words) X 0.4

The resulting figure is the Gunning–Fox index: a ready measure of the approximate number of years of schooling required to be able to read the text. Most academic writing results in a score between 10 and 17. Scores greater than 17 are usually reported as 17 – considered to be post-graduate reading level. Easy reading scores 6–10. The average reading level is 9.
Typical Fog Index scores include these:

Magazines, TV guides	– 6
Reader's Digest	– 8
Many novels	– 10
The Times, The Guardian	– 14
Academic papers in scientific journals	– 15–20

There are many such tests which are easy to find on the internet. Some example sites are:

- http://www.literacytrust.org.uk/campaign/SMOG.html
- http://www.tasc.ac.uk/depart/media/staff/ls/modules/MED1140/Fog.htm
- http://www.usingenglish.com/glossary/readability-test.html
- http://www.healthsystem.virginia.edu/internet/health-education/read.cfm
- http://www.juicystudio.com/fog/
- http://www.sharedlearning.org.uk/fog_index.htm (helpful for those with English as a second language)

Figure 5.1 Amended information for children (supplementary to parental information)

Hello. My name is _____

I work at _____ University.

I am making a video about nurses who look after children.

If you want to be in it I will video the nurses when they are looking after you.

I will ask your Mum or Dad if they think it's OK for you to be in the video.

You don't have to be in it.

You can say no – that's OK.

If you want to be in the video and then change your mind - that's OK too.

If there is anything you are not sure about just ask me.

Proxy consent

When children are unable to determine what is in their best interests, parents are normally the best alternative decision-makers. In situations where the planned research participants are children under the care of the social services, special care needs to be taken to be sure that decisions are taken by the appropriate legal guardian. Even being sure that a parent has parental rights and responsibilities may not be so straightforward under the terms of the Children Act 1989. Additional factors come into play if the mother is herself less than 16 years of age. In this case she must

Figure 5.2 Information sheet for parents of a child to be included in a study (With the permission of Joan Livesley)

Working with children

An invitation to children and young people who use hospital services

Information for parents and Carers

[insert photograph]

Who am I?

My name is Joan Livesley, I work at the University of Salford and am a children's nurse. I am currently undertaking research to find out what helps children and young people feel safe in hospital and what makes them feel unsafe or insecure. I have previous experience of doing research but this project is being supervised by Dr. Tony Long. Tony is also employed by the University of Salford and is also a children's nurse.

Why do you want to speak to my child?

Your hospital consultant has given permission for me to ask you if I can approach your child to see if they would like to be involved in this research project.

This work is about undertaking a research project in partnership with children who have been in hospital and are likely to go into hospital in the future.

As your child has been in hospital in the last 12 months and is likely to go into hospital again I would like to invite them to participate in the study.

What do you hope to find out?

I hope to find what children think about being in hospital, what helps to make them feel safe and what makes them feel unsafe?

What will you do with the findings?

The findings will be used to produce a tool kit that can be used by people who work in hospital to create an environment that helps children feel safe

What would my child's involvement be?

Initially, this would involve joining a focus group of about 9 other children to talk about their experiences of being in hospital. The focus groups will take place at the hospital in a comfortable room not on

the ward. Focus groups are useful as they help children think about what others have said and they can be fun.

If your child would rather talk to me on a one to one basis then that is fine as well and I can arrange for a 1 to 1 interview at a time and place convenient to you.

Will you write down what they say?

I may, but with your child's permission I would like to tape record the conversation

Will you do anything else besides talking to my child?

Yes, I will use games and other fun activities to help the children tell me about their experiences of being in hospital. The activities will be age appropriate and children will only have to join in those they wish to.

How long will the focus group last?

Between 1 hour and 90 minutes. This is to give the

children time to settle down before we start to talk.

Can I stay with my child?

Yes, of course, and you are welcome to bring your partner or other children if you wish.

Who will find out what my child has said?

I will write about what your child has said and I will give presentations to hospital staff and at professional conferences to make sure that their views and opinions are heard by as many people who work in hospital and train others to work in hospital as possible. However, your child will be given a different name so that nobody can identify them as an individual.

Does my child have to take part?

No, even if you give permission for your child to take part but they do not wish to no pressure will be put on them to do so.

What happens next?

If you are willing for your child to take part, please

pass on the children's invitation sent with this information asking them if they would like to take part. If they agree then both of you should sign the consent form (children can choose to place the sticker enclosed in the pack on the form as well as or instead of signing the form). When you have done this, please return the form to me in the stamped self addressed envelope. I will then contact you with details of when the group interviews will take place or arrange for a 1 to 1 interview.

Will our information remain confidential?

Yes, all children and families who agree to take part will be given different names in any written or verbal presentation. All research data will be kept in a secure locked archive and all personal information will be treated as confidential. However, if any child tells me that someone is causing them harm I will pass this information on to others.

The research tapes, notes and transcripts will be kept for 10 years. At the end of this time your child may have their tape returned or I can arrange to have it destroyed.

What will happen when the research is complete?

I will write to you and let you know what I have found out, you will be invited to meetings of parents, children and hospital staff to discuss the findings. You will also be invited to join events where the findings will be disseminated to others.

Can I or my children become more involved in the research?

Yes, I am looking for adult and child volunteers to join the study review group. This group will meet at least once per year; review the research processes and the findings as they emerge. If you or your child would like to become involved with this work, please let me know.

What if I am unsure, who do I contact for more information?

You can speak to your Doctor or Nurse or contact me on 0161 295 7018 or by email at j.livesley@salford.ac.uk

Thank you for taking the time to read this information leaflet

Joan Livesley (to be signed by hand)

Joan Livesley RSCN, BSc., MA
University of Salford
Allerton Building, Room C603
Frederick Road,
Salford
M30 0NN

be deemed to be 'Gillick competent' (see Chapter 4) to exercise parental rights and responsibilities in deciding about the child's participation in research. Those with authority to make proxy decisions on behalf of a child must do so only on the basis of adequate information and being satisfied that non-therapeutic research (that is, research which will not offer any benefit to the individual child) is not against the best interests of the child and will impose only a minimal burden (Department of Health 2001a).

It is not only children, however, who may be represented by a proxy. Older people (perhaps with dementia), people with learning disabilities, and people with mental-health problems may also have their interests represented by a third party. This may be formalised as through an advanced directive or legal advocate, or someone holding responsibility through the nature of their post. It is wise for researchers to ensure the validity of claims to act as a proxy before accepting them at face value.

Acting in the individual's best interests

An individual's best interests are not limited to what may benefit them most medically. Their cultural, religious or spiritual values are also important, as well as their chosen lifestyle and preferences expressed while competent. It is vital that researchers consider the best interests only of the individual whose participation is sought. The interests of family, society or a health professional discipline must be subordinated to this. Whenever possible the view of an independent third party should be sought, and the views and reflections of those who are close to the individual should also be taken into account.

Recording evidence

The Department of Health is very clear on the nature of a signed consent form (Box 5.4) whether for medical treatment or for research purposes (Department of Health 2001b).

> *Legally, it makes no difference whether patients sign a form to indicate their consent, or whether they give consent orally or even non-verbally... A consent form is only a record, not proof that genuine consent has been given.*

Nevertheless, it is important for such documentary evidence as does exist to have been completed properly and then stored securely. The length of time for which materials must be stored varies, but local and legal requirements will need to be identified and met. The guidance from COREC is that copies

Box 5.4 The COREC standardised consent form

(Form to be on headed paper)

Centre Number:

Study Number:

Patient Identification Number for this trial:

CONSENT FORM

Title of Project:

Name of Researcher:

Please initial box

1. I confirm that I have read and understand the
   information sheet dated ....
   (version ....) for the above study. I have had
   the opportunity to consider the information, ask
   questions and have had these answered satisfactorily.

2. I understand that my participation is voluntary and
   that I am free to withdraw at any time, without
   giving any reason, without my medical care or legal
   rights being affected.

3. I understand that relevant sections of any of my
   medical notes and data collected during the study,
   may be looked at by responsible individuals from
   [company name], from regulatory authorities or from
   the NHS Trust, where it is relevant to my taking part
   in this research. I give permission for these individuals
   to have access to my records.

4. I agree to my GP being informed of my participation
   in the study.

5. I agree to take part in the above study.

_____   _____   _____
Name of Patient   Date   Signature

_____   _____   _____
Name of Person taking consent   Date   Signature
(if different from researcher)

_____   _____   _____
Researcher   Date   Signature

When completed, 1 for patient; 1 for researcher site file; 1
(original) to be kept in medical notes

should be held by the participant and the researcher, and a third copy placed in the medical records where appropriate. The evidence should include statements that due information has been provided and understood, and that the individual has agreed voluntarily to participate; in addition, there should be a brief statement of agreement to the requirement of the study.

Undertaking research without consent

It is perfectly possible to conduct research secretly. However, to do so in a way that avoids serious harms can be challenging and individualises the responsibility for any unfortunate outcomes. Clarke (2004) argues that covert research which he undertook in a secure mental health unit would have been impossible by more open means. He suggests that the custodial culture in that setting would have prohibited more open study. This meant, however, that he alone shouldered the responsibility for decisions he made in this study and he admits that his relations with the unit concerned were very much soured in the aftermath. Clarke's defence of his covert approach is well-articulated and disarmingly honest. This can reassure us that, in the absence of formal ethical approval, he acted with sound motives even if the means remain questionable. Certainly, investigators and their supervisors should not ordinarily avoid formal approval mechanisms, as this could be fraught with dangers, both to potential research participants and to the researchers themselves. In contrast, a key example of research undertaken without consent yet certainly meeting ethical requirements is the Unlinked Anonymous Prevalence Monitoring Programme (detailed in Chapter 4), which studies the distribution of undiagnosed infection in the population of the UK (Health Protection Agency 2005).

Ensuring continued consent

Most authorities agree that gaining consent should be viewed as an on-going process rather than a one-off event. This may be achieved by formal means (with planned review dates) or informally by verbal checks ('Are you still OK about me taking an extra 5 ml of blood for the research study?'). A balance should be sought, however, between unnecessarily causing concern to the participant ('Why do they keep asking me that? Maybe something is wrong?'), and offering the opportunity for someone who is already genuinely regretting their agreeing to participate. The skill to gauge this balance ought to be held by most health professionals who deal on a daily basis with patients and clients.

Completing the process in the case of implied or delayed consent

While it is acceptable to commence data collection in some cases when subjects are unable to express a choice about participation, this choice must be offered as soon as possible after the individual becomes able to consider the issues and make a decision. Their decision about the use of existing data must then be respected.

PRESERVING CONFIDENTIALITY

A second issue of vital importance in respecting the individual as a research participant is safeguarding their privacy. A number of standard techniques are advised in order to protect confidentiality. Storing data securely (and usually separate from personal details of the sample), the use of pseudonyms to represent the identity of participants (protecting their anonymity), and routines for the disposal of material at the end of the study are all employed.

The Data Protection Act 1988

Arrangements to preserve confidentiality are now affected by the need to comply with the terms of the Data Protection Act 1998. This came into force on 1st March 2000, replacing the Data Protection Act 1984 and repealing large sections of the Access to Health Records Act 1990. The new act extended the protection of personal information to all records whether physical (paper based) or electronic. The act refers to the 'processing' of data, which includes the collection, use, disclosure, destruction and holding of data. Eight data-protection principles are expressed to which organisations processing personal data must adhere. Data must be:

- fairly and lawfully processed
- processed for limited purposes
- adequate, relevant and not excessive
- accurate
- kept no longer than necessary
- processed in accordance with individuals' rights
- kept secure
- given adequate protection if transferred to non-EEA countries.

Sensitive data (including data on a person's ethnic origins, religious beliefs, political opinions, health, sexual life and any criminal history) is subject to additional requirements. Additional information may be found at the website of the Information Commissioner.[1]

Disclosure to a third party

It has become traditional in much nursing and health research to assure research participants and organisations of the confidentiality of the data collected. However, researchers need to be aware that in a research context (as in a clinical one) they may become privileged with information of great importance, for example in a criminal matter. However, when personal safety or the protection of vulnerable people is an issue, confidentiality cannot be considered an absolute duty. This should also, however, be made clear to participants. Declarations by participants that suggest the potential for harm to themselves or third parties should prompt the researcher seriously to consider divulging the essential information to an appropriate authority or professional.

This stance is supported by the famous Tarasoff judgement. In this case a psychiatric patient, Prosenjit Poddar, told a psychologist during a formal therapy session that he planned to kill Tatiana Tarasoff (another student who had spurned his advances to her). The therapist maintained confidentiality, but Poddar did, indeed, kill Tarasoff 2 months later. The minority opinion on the case was that warning an intended victim in such cases would offer little benefit to society (since the authorities could do little to protect against the many empty threats that are made in this way); would frustrate the success of psychiatric treatment (by destroying the trust between patient and doctor or therapist, resulting in the loss of liberty for many harmless individuals); and would increase violence by causing individuals to be hesitant to reveal their violent fantasies or plans. (Having no professional outlet they would be more likely to act out their feelings.) However, the majority opinion recognised the right to privacy in the professional–client relationship, but maintained that doctors and therapists owe a duty not only to the client but also to the intended victim. The requirement to disclose information of a serious threat to a third party was aptly framed in the pronouncement that: 'The protective privilege ends where the public peril begins.'

---

[1] http://www.informationcommissioner.gov.uk/cms/DocumentUploads/Data%20Protection%20ACT%20Fact%20V2.pdf

The outcome of this is that confidentiality should normally be maintained in a research study, but if information is discovered that implies a serious risk to a third party, the public, or even the participant themselves (notably if the participant is a child), then controlled disclosure to an appropriate authority is required.

Anonymity

One of the more common (and sometimes effective) ways to protect confidentiality is to anonymise details of participants and organisations involved in a study. Pseudonyms are used for people, while institutions and organisations may be referred to only in vague terms ('a general hospital in the North of England'). As an effort to protect participants, this is of course commendable. However, closer review of the phenomenon and comparison with approaches applied in other fields of investigation suggests some lack of consistency. We have argued elsewhere (Johnson 2004, Johnson & Long 2006) that in historical research or in investigative journalism (both aimed at enhancing the general good through rigorous review of data) it is appropriate and sometimes essential to provide accurate details of participants and to offer significant personal details relating to the case. 'Fly-on-the-wall' exposé documentaries transmit still and video images with full sound (and often subtitles) to the public and the authorities of poor practices in hospitals and public establishments (nurseries, care homes, police stations). No consent is sought and no information provided before data collection. Confidentiality is simply not an issue. Yet similar activity in a declared research project would be instantly condemned. We might wonder how the display to millions of television viewers of patients becoming distressed through bad news of a loved-one or their own diagnosis for the sake of general interest may be seen to be acceptable while it can be so difficult to have research interviews approved by ethics and governance committees.

Many television documentaries about health care are in some ways analogous to research and contain extremely personal information about named respondents, but provided the individuals concerned give consent to the publication of these data, the programme is screened. Further thought is needed about the relative risks and benefits, and the validity of the comparison between investigative or documentary journalism and research. Nevertheless, it is a requirement for researchers to adopt a different set of rules to those applied to journalism, and, for the moment at least, the convention of rendering research participants and organisations anonymous in reports is probably wise in most cases. Where identities are to be revealed this should be agreed in writing in advance of any publication or report.

Storing data safely

A principal strategy for health and nursing research is the collection of data about people. The data may include personal, biographical and demographic information that should normally be used for this purpose only. Some research methods, such as focus groups, can mean that people are aware of the responses of others. For this reason, people need to be aware of the implications and of any ground-rules that information so gained is kept private to the group. Data of a novel or non-standard nature may include video images and voices; still photography; computerised patient records; paintings, sculpture, drama and other forms of expression; and human tissues. The processing and safe, confidential storage of such media can present something of a challenge. However, their use is not, of itself, unethical. Indeed, a study may have greater moral force the more appropriate and convincing the methods used. As we have argued elsewhere, probably too many researchers use the semi-structured interview as the default method (Long & Johnson 2000). Guidance which is specific to the use of video and audio recording with patients as research subjects is provided by the General Medical Council (2002).

Disposal of materials

Data must not only be stored securely but also disposed of in an equally secure manner. Many think that data used for one purpose should not, without permission, be used for any other. It seems reasonable to suggest that research participants should certainly be aware of any such other uses that might be proposed. However, we suggest that it may be unwise to underestimate the value of data, suitably anonymised and carefully stored; it may offer great benefit in the future. It is even conceivable that 'routine' data could become of major significance to historians. Of course it is important that people are generally aware, where possible, that it might be used to support research in due course or on more than one occasion. Prior to data destruction, a full appraisal should be made of the risks and benefits attaching to the data. Consent to use images (particularly of children) has received much attention in recent years. Many authorities now offer guidelines on processes for collection, storage and use of such sensitive material. One good example of this may be found on the website of Hampshire County Council (Hampshire County Council 2005).

It is not uncommon for data to be returned to participants, perhaps when diaries have been used to record reflections and experiences. Such documents can be both helpful and of great emotional value to the individuals who composed them. The use of hand-delivery or special postal arrangements to ensure safe transfer between researcher and participant will be required. This can be more difficult when data from more than one respondent is included in a single item (perhaps an interview with a group of young people or a number of family members), but the rules to govern this should be agreed before data collection starts.

The means of destroying data depends upon the nature of the material. Computer disks can be physically destroyed after files have been permanently deleted; though stringent efforts need to be made to ensure that other copies have not been retained. Sound processes throughout the study for recording and controlling the number and location of copies of files is essential to this. Audio tapes can be passed through a device that incorporates a strong magnetic field to erase any recorded data permanently. Paper-based data should be shredded and disposed of through a reputable recycler.

MEASURES TO ADDRESS THE NEEDS OF SPECIFIC GROUPS

The role of consumer groups in protecting the welfare and best interests of their members has become increasingly important in the last decade. These exist for many sub-populations, such as those with mental illness, older people, or those with specific medical conditions. INVOLVE, a national group funded by the Department of Health, promotes and supports active public involvement in NHS, public health and social care research.

> We believe that the active involvement of the public in the research process leads to research that is more relevant to people and is more likely to be used. Research which reflects the needs and views of the public, is more likely to produce results that can be used to improve practice in health and social care. [2]

---

[2] http://www.invo.org.uk

INVOLVE and other groups with similar aims provide guidance for researchers as well as for the public, and it is wise for researchers to check for resources on the relevant web sites.

Mental illness

Just as with other groups of potential recruits to research studies, individuals suffering from mental illness may present particular difficulties for the researcher in terms of ensuring valid consent and establishing the individual's wishes as well as their best interests. Of course, the range of severity of mental-health problems and the degree of competence enjoyed by individuals varies greatly, so to consider 'those with mental illness' as a homogenous group is a serious mistake. Most people with a mental-health problem are able to respond competently to requests for them to participate in research. Some may need help and support from family, carers or health professionals to do so, and yet others may be simply unable to engage actively in the process. The Medical Research Council issued guidance in 1993 on 'The ethical conduct of research with the mentally incapacitated' though this has been superseded in Scotland by the introduction of the Adults with Incapacity (Scotland) Act 2000. While now rather dated, a number of key principles remain valid:

- Individuals who are unable to give valid consent should not be included in research unless it relates directly to their condition and the required knowledge could not be gained from persons who are able to give consent.
- The inclusion of an incompetent individual should be subject to the agreement of an independent authority that the research is in their best interests and their welfare has been safeguarded.
- The individual should not object or appear to object to inclusion in either words or actions (Medical Research Council 1993).

Goffman (1968) drew attention to the way in which individuals in many care environments may, sociologically speaking, lose the status normally accorded to competent adults. By this he means that by virtue of a debilitating and stigmatising form of behaviour they, for example the mentally ill, lose their normal rights and privileges. Modern approaches to research in mental health (as with research in child health) emphasise partnership between researchers and patients as research subjects. Recent developments in research with people with mental health problems in England include the creation of the Mental Health Research Network.[3] This is designed to improve the quality of mental-health research in England by acting as a resource for researchers, carers and people with mental-health problems who may consider participating in research. The initiative includes a 'Service User Research Group England' (SURGE): 'a national network set up to support mental health service users and people from universities and NHS trusts, as they work together on mental health research.'[4] It is to be expected that SURGE will be a key resource for researchers seeking guidance on good practice in research in this field. Other sources of guidance exist, though not always specific to the UK.[5]

Older people

It is tempting to assume that older people are automatically vulnerable to inappropriate clinical or research interventions, yet the majority of health-care recipients *are* older people and this trend will continue. Although it may sometimes be more convenient, excluding people from research on the grounds of age alone is not equitable and constitutes ageism. Department of Health guidance on this is that, as with other groups in society, there is a need for research in order to advance treatment and care for older people. Age is of no consequence at all if an individual is competent; they have the absolute right to decide whether or not to participate. However, the small number of older people who are not completely competent require protection. Therapeutic research may be carried out using incompetent older people as research subjects if it is in their best interest to participate, normally because they stand to receive more effective treatment from doing so. Non-therapeutic research may also be acceptable so long as the individual's interests are not jeopardised. However, as with other groups, incapacitated older people should not be included in studies if it is possible to conduct the research with people who have full capacity (competence) (Department of Health 2001b).

Other groups

A particular difficulty arises in relation to the 'very ill' where practical difficulties can be met in obtaining meaningful informed

---

[3] http://www.mhrn.info/about.html
[4] http://www.mhrn.info/surge.html
[5] For example: The National Alliance for the Mentally Ill (NAMI). http://www.nami.org/research/participating.html

consent. Many important studies have been undertaken with precisely these difficulties. Jane Seymour (2001) undertook participant observation in intensive care units focusing her attention particularly on those patients that seemed to be at the end of life. She deals in some detail (pp. 24–26) with the delicate on-going negotiation of consent with staff and patients' relatives that she undertook. Such work requires tact, sensitivity, integrity and hard work: all necessary qualities in good research.

The same applies to other groups that might require extra efforts and resources to reach, but that should not be excluded inappropriately from studies. Minority ethnic populations are sometimes difficult to involve in research, especially where there are language and cultural differences. For this reason sensitive efforts should be made to include people with such backgrounds where possible, since everyone should have the opportunity to take part in and potentially benefit from research (Gunaratnam 2003). This applies both to individuals and to whole ethnic, age, or gender groups.

CONCLUSION

Ensuring the ethical conduct of a study requires the active consideration of a number of issues by the principal investigator throughout the life of a study. Key principles include the identification of potential risks and benefits to participants, judging their competence to make a valid decision about participation, providing adequate information in a suitable format, and then acting to preserve the welfare of participants during and after the research.

REFERENCES

Clarke L (2004) Real-world ethics and nursing research: a response to Martin Johnson. NT Research 9(5), 389–391.

Consumers for Ethics in Research (1994) Spreading the word on research – or – patient information: how can we get it better? CERES, London.

Consumers for Ethics in Research (2002) Involving people who speak little or no English in health care research: information for investigators. CERES, London.

Department of Health (2001a) Seeking consent: working with children. DH, London.

Department of Health (2001b) Seeking consent: working with older people. DH, London.

General Medical Council (2002) Making and using visual and audio recordings of patients. GMC, London.

Glaser B, Strauss A (1965) Awareness of dying, Aldine, Chicago.
Goffman E (1968) Asylums, Penguin, Harmondsworth.
Gunaratnam Y (2003) Researching "race" and ethnicity, Sage, London.
Hampshire County Council (2005) Using images of people: photographs, videos and webcams.
Health Protection Agency (2005) The Unlinked Anonymous Prevalence Monitoring Programme. HPA, London.
INVOLVE (2004) A guide to actively involving young people in research:for researchers, research commissioners and managers. INVOLVE, Eastleigh.
Johnson M (2004) Real world ethics and nursing research. NT Research 9(4), 251–261.
Johnson M, Long T (2006) Research ethics. In: Gerrish K, Lacey A(eds) The research process in nursing, 5th edn. Blackwells, London.
Lawton J (2000) The dying process: patients' experiences of palliative care, Routledge, London.
Long T, Johnson M (2000) Research in Nurse Education Today: Do we meet our aims and scope? Nurse Education Today 22(1), 85–93.
Medical Research Council (1993) The ethical coduct of research on the mentally incapacitated. MRC, London.
Seymour J (2001) Critical moments – death and dying in critical care, Open University Press, Buckingham.
Stockwell F (1972, 1984) The unpopular patient, Croom Helm, London.

LEGAL REFERENCES
Tarasoff v Regents of the University of California. S. Ct. of CA, 1976 17 Cal.3d 425

6 Criticising research from an ethical point of view

Martin Johnson

INTRODUCTION

Despite a good deal of progress in the evaluation of research protocols by the various bodies and committees charged with this duty, it is still rare to find published any detailed critique of research studies from an ethical point of view. One might even assume that getting ethical clearance, and certainly having work peer reviewed and published, guarantees that the research has been conducted according to well-recognised ethical standards.

Such an assumption is false. On the one hand, most procedures for ethical scrutiny are prospective. That is, the reviewers and committees examine paperwork stating what researchers *intend* to do, rather than what they are *actually* doing or have done. In other cases, researchers choose to avoid ethics committees and other approval mechanisms. They may believe that these procedures will prevent, obstruct or delay research that they believe is in the wider public interest, or they may convince themselves that labelling their investigation as 'audit' or 'evaluation' will avoid these potentially difficult examinations.

Historically, researchers tended to assume both that their work was important and that their integrity was sufficient to avoid harms. Experienced researchers in other disciplines, from which many nurses and other health professionals borrowed their methods, tended to assume that they had a natural right to collect data in the interests of society and the furtherance of knowledge. Most notorious of these were American sociologist Laud Humphreys (1975) who secretly studied the promiscuous sexual behaviour of gay men in public places such as toilets, and psychologist Stanley Milgram (1974) who engaged volunteers to 'electrocute' research participants in a laboratory experiment in obedience to authority.

It is hardly surprising, therefore, that British nurse Dan Jones (1975) undertook a large observational study of unconscious patients in general hospital wards in which the consent of the patients or their relatives was simply not discussed. The permission of managers and consultants was then seen to be adequate. In this important study Jones and his colleague decided, for example, not to intervene even when a nurse was observed to tube-feed a patient with liquid close to boiling point and which made the syringe too hot to touch. They generally took the view that as scientists their responsibility was to report what they saw rather than to prevent harms at the time (Johnson 2004).

In this chapter I identify questions that may be asked in the examination of the ethical conduct of health care research. I then use this 'checklist' of important questions with a number of different, but largely influential studies to illustrate how the questions can promote discussion of key issues. Of course the checklist could also be applied to any study.

QUESTIONS TO ASK ABOUT RESEARCH CONDUCT

In this next section I will illustrate a framework of key questions (Box 6.1) that arise loosely from the theories discussed in Chapter 3 and try to show how this can allow useful debate of issues raised by studies and lessons that can be learned.

It is important to recognise that, particularly in journal articles, the level of detail required to answer all these questions in depth may not be available. In longer reports such as theses or reports to commissioners, however, certainly most of this might be expected. Theses are more likely to provide theoretical justifications; research reports to public bodies are more likely to report just bare facts.

1. What were the aims of the study? How important were they and why?

Humphreys (1975) undertook to study gay men secretly in public toilets in sex acts such as fellatio. He negotiated the role of 'watchqueen', a person who keeps a look-out for park wardens and the police. He subsequently (having got the subjects' addresses from a police computer) undertook a door-to-door survey to get the essential demographic data. He did much to raise awareness of homosexual behaviour about which most heterosexuals knew very little, and changed attitudes about exactly which part or level of society such people came from: all parts and all levels. Though it was not one of his aims, he raised awareness of the tricks that social researchers sometimes use to get their data and their PhD.

Box 6.1 Questions to ask about ethical issues in a research study

1. What were the aims of the study? How important were they and why?
2. Who undertook the study and how did their background prepare them?
3. Who supervised or monitored the study?
4. What sort of ethical approval was given, if any?
5. What information were participants given and how readable and accurate was this?
6. What checks were made to ensure that consent was given and remained in force?
7. What opportunities were given for participants to withdraw?
8. How were issues of power between researcher and respondents dealt with?
9. Were any social groups excluded, and if so how powerful was the justification?
10. Were participants deprived of a known helpful intervention and if so, on what grounds?
11. What risks/harms were associated with the study? Were these acceptable in the context of the potential benefits?
12. What benefits might arise from the study? Who was likely to benefit?
13. Did the effort made to disseminate the study outcomes to all concerned match the promises made?

(Adapted from Johnson and Long (2005), and reprinted with permission)

Humphreys argued that the aims of his study were to improve the lot of homosexuals in American society, but he was roundly criticised on the grounds that he infringed human freedoms, invaded privacy, risked his participants' reputations and even that he studied an area so private that it should never be studied (Warwick 1973). Even though Humphreys' work might have helped in a long process of raising awareness of homosexual oppression and developing gay rights, from a human-rights perspective he can be heavily criticised for the above reasons. It is difficult to imagine such a study being approved by the health and social research bureaucracy today. However, from the consequential perspective no participant was directly harmed and a good deal of benefit was gained. This was chiefly public awareness of gay lifestyles and a greater examination by the sociological community of its methods and practices.

2. Who undertook the study and how did their background prepare them?

Burden (1998) chose to study the delivery of hospital midwifery care, examining in particular how bed curtains were used and issues of privacy. She gained ethical approval although, as I have indicated above, from the journal article it is not clear how much of her research strategy, which included elements of covert observation, was clear to the approval committee. She observed the strategies that women used to preserve, as much as possible, their privacy in the ward environment. Indeed, it becomes clear that the midwives were finding that the women were too adept at keeping the curtains closed to exclude the midwives from their traditional clear view of the women in the ward.

Writing, arguably, from a feminist perspective, Burden is reflexively alive to the paradox in her study, that she had to invade privacy to some extent in order to study it (Johnson 2005), and that she had to use elements of covert observation. She argues that:

> *Covert observation was seen as appropriate if the care of the women was not compromised. In order to achieve this the role of midwife was adopted (we presume by Burden) to facilitate communication with women and promoted observation and discussion about their actions. Obviously it was inappropriate to gain consent to participate from individuals as the advantage of observing natural settings would have been lost.*
>
> (Burden 1998, p. 18)

In recent times such an approach, to collect data without even retrospective consent, would be seen as controversial. The question could be asked, 'Did the ethics committee approve this in advance?' However, our original question was about Burden's preparation for this study. First, she was a Registered Midwife, obviously able to play the role of qualified person and to judge safe practice in its context. She was presumably credible to the women and to the midwives as a participant in the setting. Second, she was at that time the head of her division at the university. According to the article front page she either undertook the study as part of, or already had a Master's degree in social research. She ought, then, to have understood some of these issues well. On balance, she was as well-prepared as anyone could be to feel comfortable in this setting, and yet to be able to examine it for important issues that her colleagues may not have had the time to study.

So far as one can judge from an article, Burden employed practical ethics to advantage, without causing anyone any particular harms, and the study is very informative.

3. Who supervised and monitored the study?

Many published studies are drawn from postgraduate theses for MA, MSc, MPhil, PhD or professional doctorate degrees. Conventions for acknowledging supervision in articles vary. In some departments the supervisor can be assumed to be the second named author, in others it may be the first-named author, especially if they enabled the study through grant acquisition or the study was just a part of a larger one of which they were in overall charge. In books it would be usual to acknowledge all those who helped in the preface, and similarly in the dissertation or thesis itself. Occasionally articles have an 'acknowledgment' at the end. Some research students choose not to acknowledge supervision in their publications.

These differences can mean that deducing the exact supervision arrangements can be complicated. More and more, university and public-service departments have quite rigorous arrangements for monitoring student progress. This ought to mean that work undertaken in these settings may be assumed to meet certain minimum standards. Whilst this might hold true in some cases, the level of day-to-day supervision that is possible is low. Supervisors generally rely on researchers reporting problems and discussing them rather than actually being in the field and monitoring personally. This means that individual researchers need to make practical ethical decisions on the conduct of their study and that issues that cannot be foreseen at the planning stage rely on the personal integrity of the researcher for a sound resolution. Ethics review committees in both the health services and universities require 'reports' of progress to be completed, but this could scarcely be described as close supervision.

Effectively, then, the fact that a study was undertaken within an organisational framework, for a well-known funding agency, or in a university, may give *some* reassurance that major ethical problems that could have been foreseen would have been discussed and solutions prepared. This does not guarantee that these solutions would appeal to everyone, however.

A particular difficulty arises in relation to the 'very ill' where practical difficulties can be met in obtaining meaningful informed consent. Many important studies have been undertaken with precisely these difficulties obtaining. Jane Seymour (2001) undertook participant observation in intensive care units focusing her attention particularly on patients who seemed to be at the end of life. It might be said that her respondents were extremely vulnerable. It was not only the patients and their relatives that were vulnerable in this challenging and complex environment, but also, arguably, the nurses and other health-care staff, given that Seymour was trying to study their behaviour in the context of the very ill and the dying. She reminds us that recent well-publicised cases had put nurses in the spotlight because certain individuals had been found to be abusively endangering patients. She gained approval from the local research ethics committee, but clearly feels that the most important 'ethical approval' for her was gained from the people she would be engaged in studying or those who cared about them. She deals in some detail (Seymour 2001, pp. 24–26) with the delicate on-going negotiation of consent with staff and patients' relatives that she undertook. Such work requires tact, sensitivity, integrity and hard work: all necessary qualities in good research. In addition, Seymour points out that she was supervised by David Clark, an eminent social researcher in this field and that she gained support from her colleagues in an experienced palliative-care research group.

Whilst she notes that critically ill unconscious patients cannot consent personally, and that 'proxy' consent by relatives has no legal status, this did not mean that she felt she had behaved unethically. Rather, the important insights she has disseminated and the efforts she put into securing the agreement of those concerned who could consent, and the quality of her academic supervision can lead us to conclude that she has done little if any harm and a lot of good. As importantly, she debates her own ethical conduct for other researchers to learn from and discuss in the context of their own studies, rather than merely avoiding the challenges faced by this environment.

4. What sort of ethical approval was gained, if any?

In health research it has become much less common for studies to be undertaken without any formal ethics approval. Occasionally, however, researchers or approval bodies feel that it is not necessary because their study does not qualify as 'research', such as work classified as audit or evaluation. Clarke (1996) undertook a covert study of a mental-health setting because he felt that, whilst the study was important, the hospital management would be unlikely to consent (Clarke 2004, Johnson 2004). Having been criticised for failing to gain consent from those studied, he makes a plausible case that in certain circumstances, experienced researchers ought to be able to study certain contexts without local consent, especially where professional power might be abused. In this case the setting was a secure mental-health unit, in some ways analogous to a prison. He does not deny that this has its risks, not least being unwelcome in that type of setting in the future, but on the balance of outcomes he feels more good was done than harm. It is for others to judge, but researchers need to tread this path carefully and only with full support in other respects, such as the approval of a sponsor or university supervision team.

5. What information were participants given? How readable and accurate was this?

Individuals who are able to consider what participation will involve should be able to decide whether or not to take part in a study. Full and readily comprehensible information should be provided and software is now available to evaluate its readability (Johnson & Long 2005). Other standard tests of readability based on sentence length and other criteria are also available (see Chapter 5). Whilst journal articles will rarely be so detailed, theses, books and full reports for funding bodies should contain examples of the information given. It may be important to evaluate the degree to which information meets the needs of minorities or people who may be involved but whose first language is not that of the researchers (Gunaratnam 2003, Royal College of Nursing Research Society 2003). Whilst such considerations might seem methodological, the question of whether studies meet the needs of all in society whose interests are of concern is clearly an ethical one.

6. What checks were made to ensure that consent was given and remained in force?

In Seymour's (2001) study of the dying in intensive care units (discussed earlier), she regularly reminded participants of her research role and re-negotiated this as days went by. On the other hand, reminding respondents to excess can lead to nervousness that their involvement is more harmful than it really is. Where a clear record of consent has been obtained then researchers should be mindful of any reason that this might have changed. In some studies, a clinical deterioration might lead to future exclusion of a respondent, but it would be wrong to assume this in all cases. As Seymour (2001) and Lawton (2000) illustrate, it may be more important to study the very ill, but most properly when this has been discussed with those concerned and agreed in advance. In most studies of an experimental nature, it may be clearer to what individuals have consented and under precisely what conditions the study may be undertaken.

7. What opportunities were given for participants to withdraw?

Increasingly it is seen as good practice to allow potential research participants a period during which to consider their involvement rather than being confronted with the information and a consent form at one and the same moment in which they must decide. Wherever practicable, information should be available in advance of recruitment and data collection, but there will be many circumstances in which this is impractical. For example, in a study of men with acute chest pain White and Johnson (2000) needed to observe and, where possible, interview men and their partners within hours of admission to hospital once their pain had moderated. In this case several days' notice was impossible, but patients had the option to be excluded from the dataset if they later felt uncomfortable with inclusion.

Health and social care organisations (for example casualty departments (Moskop et al. 2005)) can be incredibly complex with hundreds of people passing through or being present transiently for a few moments. People undertaking studies that employ covert methods or even which openly study such complex social situations may need to recognise that neither gaining true informed consent nor providing an opportunity to withdraw may be possible. Some people from whom data are collected in these situations may never be able to give consent. This needs to be considered but should not be seen as a reason for the avoidance of such situations. Other mechanisms exist for safeguarding privacy, such as individual and organisational anonymity, and use of pseudonyms. It may be possible to gain consent from some people, and from the consequential perspective, some consent is better than none. It might provide an indication of the degree to which those who could not be consulted might also feel comfortable.

8. How were issues of power between researcher and respondents dealt with?

It seems to be very common for academics of many disciplines to study their own students, staff, or patients. Such an arrangement clearly provides a good deal of convenience to the researcher that should, however, be balanced against the very grave limitations imposed by such an approach for generalisation beyond that setting. It is particularly unfortunate when this approach is taken with methods clearly designed for wider application, such as questionnaires. A number of justifications do exist for investigating those in your own setting, however. Having undertaken the same course a few years earlier and now working as a lecturer in that department, Luker (1984) interviewed her students on an undergraduate nursing degree programme about some of their experiences, notably the difficulties and stigma they experienced as being 'different' to the more traditionally trained hospital-based students.

More recently, at least one graduate of that same programme, Elliott, undertook a study of 14 undergraduates at the different university department where she now works (Pearcey & Elliott 2004). These investigators used focus groups rather than individual interviews on the grounds that they might have 'intimidated some students'. Whilst they offer little detail, they were clearly concerned that their positions as staff, with the authority to mark and grade students, might coerce students, especially individually, to respond in a particular way. Pearcey and Elliott offer no evidence that their study was approved by an ethics committee, but make clear that student participation was voluntary, and the fact that a number declined illustrates that they did not feel coerced to participate. The study is typical of the way that education staff might capitalise on the opportunity to study their students by engaging in an arguably more rigorous and systematic form of evaluation that meets publication standards.

Senior staff are often engaged to study the implementation of policy and to evaluate service delivery. Done routinely this amounts to audit, but when theoretically informed and conducted with rigour and detailed analysis such activity becomes research. In a study of the implementation of a participatory decision-making system called shared governance, Williamson (2003, 2004) worked as a nurse consultant introducing change and recording, via various ethnographic methods and an action research perspective, the processes and outcomes. The study was granted ethical approval, and had the benefit of management support, but is at the margins of the degree to which personal anonymity can be maintained because of the known association of people with particular roles. Whilst the organisation chose not to remain anonymous, since its investment in the innovation was a key aspect of its policy, being so closely involved with less senior staff as participants leaves open questions about the degree to which individuals may feel little choice about their involvement in such a study. Williamson managed this situation by holding regular open meetings where staff could express their feelings without recrimination, and, to some extent, enabling colleagues to take some ownership of the study. Whilst one might harbour slight concerns about any particularly vulnerable staff, it is important to remember that such studies are unlikely to do serious harm and that health service staff at a professional level ought to have the social skills to deal directly with researchers if they have any concerns, and resolve them.

Seal et al. (2000) note that, occasionally, researchers in the sexual behaviour field get involved in personal relationships with research participants. Whilst he was a postgraduate PhD student, Dingwall (1977) undertook an influential study of health visitor training of the time. In addition to a detailed review of the history and social policy leading to the training of health visitors of the day, Dingwall (not otherwise a health professional) undertook open fieldwork for a year as participant observer, sharing many lessons, coffee breaks and social events with the students on the course. Beginning a fashion for self-disclosure, Dingwall explains that he found himself becoming involved with one of the respondents to the extent that he felt this might compromise the quality of his data and analysis. He describes his dilemma as the libidinal dimension of ethnography and shares his concern that he might have in some way exploited his position as a (male) postgraduate in relation to the (female) health visitors. All these years later I think he can be assured that health visitors probably are not so in awe of PhD students as he might have thought. As Harris (1985) argues, sex is only wrong when there is 'violation, exploitation, the infliction of harm, pain (or) suffering'. Only his partner can decide whether these were present: somehow I think not, since they later married.

It is inevitable that in many research situations with patients, the knowledge and position of the researcher may enable exploitation. Frankly, a close intimate relationship with a research participant who is vulnerable in the added respect of being a patient is likely to be seen as professional misconduct. Such matters are unlikely to appear in publications, however honest the researcher.

9. Were any social groups excluded? If so how powerful was the justification?

In the analysis of even recent previous work it may be unfair to be too critical of researchers who seem, with hindsight, to have excluded certain groups of respondents for what may seem, from a modern and more inclusive point of view, to be rather weak reasons. For example, Wiles et al. (2004) report a study of discharge from physiotherapy following stroke in which they followed 16 patients collecting data by qualitative methods in case studies.

> *The study participants were drawn from patients admitted to three National Health Service (NHS) acute hospital trusts in the South of England following stroke. Patients were recruited to the study through hospital physiotherapists, who identified eligible patients. The inclusion criteria were that: patients were referred for out-patient physiotherapy following the first incidence of stroke; that they had no other major medical conditions and that they were able to communicate and comprehend English. Patients over 80 years of age were excluded because of the likelihood that they would have other pre-existing conditions that would impact on treatment......Approval was granted by the Local Research Ethics Committees in which the Trusts were located.*

(Wiles 2004)

This study, undertaken by a well-qualified multi-professional team, nevertheless excluded a number of key social groups without sufficient rationale. First, patients were recruited by physiotherapists themselves, rather than researchers, so one might reasonably doubt the consistent application of inclusion criteria. Second, only patients whose condition was a first incidence were welcome in the study. Third, patients, despite already being vulnerable to stroke (which often has cardiac, diabetic, or other pre-existing pathology) were expected not to have any other major medical condition. Though questionable, these exclusions might be defensible on the grounds of reasonable comparability between treatment groups, even though nothing in the way of statistical experimental manipulation was envisaged as this was a wholly qualitative study of small groups.

Of perhaps greater concern is the fourth exclusion, of people who could not speak English. Generally in the UK those with an Asian background endure worse health and, in particular, a higher incidence of stroke (London Health Observatory 2005). Whilst Asians are the largest minority group in the UK whose older residents might not speak English, others might also have been excluded. Given the relatively small size of the study, it might have been feasible to arrange interpreters or family support. Let us at least hope that some reasonable method was found of communicating with these research-excluded non-English-speaking respondents for clinical reasons even though they did not find themselves eligible for the study.

One might assume that those studying stroke-care services might generally avoid an ageist point of view. Even less defensible, therefore, is the exclusion of the over 80s on the *assumption* that they must have pre-existing medical conditions that would impact on treatment. I see no justification for such exclusion, and more probably this reflects a prejudice of either the research team or the bureaucracy they had to satisfy to gain approval.

Whilst it is wrong to assume that all people with stroke are old, it seems completely wrong to exclude from study those who, by reason of being old, are more likely to be socially excluded in more respects than just from the study by Wiles and colleagues.

10. Were participants deprived of a known helpful intervention and if so, on what grounds?

A fundamental problem in the use of trials or experiments to compare treatments or potentially helpful interventions of any kind is that in order to make the comparison subjects are allocated to one or more groups, not all of which will receive the intervention. Often, a control group will receive no treatment, so that they can act as a benchmark to compare benefits of the new care with. This can mean that individuals are left without the benefit of a treatment known to be useful. Whilst every effort is made to avoid this situation, especially where people are threatened by serious illness, it is not always avoidable.

In order for the study to be conducted with minimum risk, enough needs to be known about each intervention for it to be considered safe. This can mean that we already know which is likely to be the most helpful intervention, but just want to do a more rigorous study to make the evidence even more certain. A good example is the celebrated study by Boore (1978): a nurse with a background as a physiologist who chose patients undergoing routine surgery. Before the operation she gave one group a special teaching session on postoperative recovery, including specific information on what to expect, breathing and stretching exercises and how to ask for analgesia. The control group just had the researcher chatting about general topics for the same period of time pre-operatively. The results quite strongly confirmed that the 'experimental' group to which Boore had given special information left hospital earlier, had lower urine steroid levels, implying they was less stressed, and suffered fewer wound infections.

It would be fatuous to imply that Boore's study was 'unethical', indeed the importance that Boore was able to attach to pre-operative information in nursing curricula as a result of this study has no doubt improved the recovery period of thousands of operative patients. Nevertheless, Boore clearly had a very strong idea that the information pack would be useful. Hayward (1975) had already shown that generally similar principles were relevant in reducing post-operative pain, and Boore's literature review makes clear that a good deal of evidence pointed to the benefits of pre-operative information. She suggests, however, that no study had at that time studied the effects of her intervention on stress levels in particular.

We may ask whether any patients were deprived of a known helpful intervention. That is a matter of judgement. We know that Boore's group of 'matched' controls was deprived of her skills, as a trained nurse teacher and physiologist, in explaining how they might best recover. If Boore is honest, she knew the intervention would be helpful: all the evidence pointed to it. But to be fair, this had not been demonstrated in the UK context with any rigour, and especially not using the biochemical analysis of urine steroid levels. Indeed, if there was any doubt at all, that might have meant that the intervention might have been harmful. Perhaps, as Mitchell (2001) has found, explaining hospital procedures in detail makes *some* people *more* anxious. Furthermore, even the matched controls still got 'routine care' which means that they were not deprived of anything the average patient might expect at that time and, therefore, just in case there was a risk attached to Boore's intervention, they were better off. In summary, the risks and benefits approach is highly relevant here. Had Boore not done the study, neither these patients nor any later would have benefited.

11. What were the risk/harms associated with the study? Were these acceptable in the context of the potential benefits?

In the study by Boore (1978) above she notes that one of her two nurse research assistants was undermining the validity of the study by failing to withhold 'sympathy and encouragement that she felt the patients needed' (Boore 1994, p. 44). Similar problems were encountered by Oakley (1990) in a study of focused community midwifery support for at risk families. Oakley found that some of the midwives in her study could not comfortably allocate at-risk families to the group which would, as controls, receive what they believed to be less help. In each of these cases those actually implementing the research study were, for the very best of reasons, undermining the scientific rigour of the study. As Watson (1996) puts it, 'the more ethical you try to be the less scientific you become' (p. 7). Nevertheless, in some cases the harm prevented may be very great indeed. Fitzsimmons and McAloon (2004) had to change the protocol of a large descriptive study of people awaiting coronary bypass surgery because, four patients having died during this waiting period, they felt it necessary to intervene where patients' clinical condition had worsened.

Whether risks and harms are appropriate will always be a judgement, and is the proper province of research ethics committees.

12. What benefits were thought possible to arise from the study? Who was likely to benefit?

Gelling (2004) carefully analyses the issues arising when doing research with patients in a vegetative state (permanently comatose). This condition, often the result of traumatic brain injury, is, he argues, one of the best known but least understood, because of the high profile of cases such as Tony Bland who was injured in a crowd crush at a European Cup football match.

Clearly such individuals cannot themselves consent to research, and even proxy consent by relatives (as was discussed by Seymour 2001) has no legal status. This means that, as with clinical treatment, any harms coming to the individual might lead to the organisation being liable. One can understand the natural reluctance to approve or recommend research with such individuals for the reason that they are obviously among the most vulnerable humans in our care. Gelling (2004) argues persuasively, however, that such an approach is just as likely to disadvantage people in a persistent vegetative state. He claims that 'it is now generally accepted that all patient groups should benefit from health and social care research' (p.7).

He shows that by not being considered eligible for participation in research, such patients are excluded from the potential for benefit. It may be important here to distinguish between benefits that may accrue to the individual (so-called therapeutic research) and those positive outcomes that might reasonably only help those with similar conditions in the future.

Gelling suggests that 'The aim of all clinical research is to improve the wellbeing and health of individuals and society' (p. 13). But a problem with this is that benefits are hard to define for such a group because in many cases the potential to improve the outcome is so poor. Moreover, it can even be argued that such individuals have no interests since they have no awareness of these. Rather, any relevant interests are those of people who care for the individual in one way or another. Research proposals need to be able to identify, at least to some extent, what such diffuse benefits might be, but also what safeguards are in place, not just at the approval time but on a continuing basis, to prevent such patients being used inappropriately.

Clearly, in most experimental studies with less dependent patients, we can safely identify possible benefits both for individuals and for either that patient group or society as a whole. In qualitative or exploratory work this can be less clear-cut, but the potential harms may be less. What is important is that both researchers and their evaluators think clearly about the benefits and risks rather than adhering to 'rules' that this or that group should not be studied.

13. Did the efforts made to disseminate the study outcomes to all concerned match the promises made?

The fact that you are reading a study in order to evaluate critically its conduct might mean the authors took some steps to disseminate their work. On the other hand, despite the promises made to respondents, that the work would possibly 'make a difference', all too often researchers write only a thesis, a report that never gets wide circulation, or an article for a relatively obscure journal. Good practice should certainly include some form of readily comprehensible summary of the main research findings for all those who may have helped, such as staff, students and service users. It might include a conference or study day in a local venue for those involved, or a website with key outcomes and issues. Ideally, researchers publish, especially larger studies, in both popular and more academic forms so that most needs are met. Certainly when examining research dissertations and theses these issues ought to be taken into account.

Many researchers may find their enthusiasm for continued engagement with a topic may wane, especially after graduation or presentation of the formal report to the funding body. Whilst breaking the promise to disseminate itself may be explainable because researchers, like any contractors, often have to bid for funds and meet regular deadlines, the long-term commitment of research participants to being studied will also deteriorate if researchers cannot be relied upon to make the most of the time, effort, invasion of privacy, and, occasionally, genuine risk of harm that participants endure.

CONCLUSION

In this chapter I have proposed a number of questions that might be asked of any research study in evaluating its conduct from a moral point of view. Whilst some questions may be more important than others, and in articles some answers may not be found, having a constructively critical attitude to the research we read will help both students and experienced researchers to clarify their own values, or basic ethical framework, and may enable explanation or even change. For example, following such criticism Clarke (2004) was able to clarify the reasoning behind his covert approach in the study of care in a forensic psychiatric unit in a way that enables understanding, if not agreement, with his approach.

The questions do not imply that any particular approach is right or wrong. Rather, in answering these questions we look for compelling reasons why, in terms of its possible benefits or unfortunate consequences, an approach is justified or not. There is no 'perfect state' of ethical probity and the relative morality of the conduct of a study will vary according to the values and ethical perspectives of the evaluators (see Chapter 3). What is important is that these arguments are more commonly in the public domain, and particularly available to those with whom we do research: the participants or subjects.

REFERENCES

Boore J (1978) Prescription for recovery. Royal College of Nursing, London.

Boore J (1994) Prescription for recovery. In: Hayward J, Boore J (eds) Research Classics from the Royal College of Nursing. Scutari, Harrow.

Burden B (1998) Privacy or help? The use of curtain positioning strategies within the maternity ward environment as a means of achieving and maintaining privacy, or as a form of signalling to peers and professionals in an attempt to seek information of support. Journal of Advanced Nursing 27: 15–23.

Clarke L (1996) Participant observation in a secure unit: care conflict and control. NT Research 1(6), 431–440.

Clarke L (2004) Real-world ethics and nursing research: A response to Martin Johnson. Journal of Research in Nursing 9(Sep), 389–391.

Dingwall R (1977) The social organisation of health visitor training. Unpublished PhD thesis, University of Aberdeen.

Fitzsimmons D, McAloon T (2004) The ethics of non-intervention in a study of patients awaiting coronary artery bypass surgery. Journal of Advanced Nursing 46(4), 395–402.

Gelling L (2004) Researching patients in the vegetative state: difficulties of studying this patient group. NT Research 9(1), 7–17.

Gunaratnam Y (2003) Researching 'race' and ethnicity: methods, knowledge and power, Sage, London.

Harris J (1985) The value of life. Routledge and Kegan Paul, London.

Hayward J (1975) Information: a prescription against pain. Royal College of Nursing, London.

Humphreys L (1975) The tearoom trade. Aldine, Chicago.

Johnson M (2004) Real world ethics and nursing research. NT Research, now Journal of Research in Nursing, 9(4), 251–261.

Johnson M (2005) Notes on the tension between privacy and surveillance in nursing. In On-Line Journal of Issues in Nursing 10(2), Manuscript 3., Vol. 2005 Kent State University, USA. www.nursingworld.org/ojin/topic27/tpc27_3.htm

Johnson M, Long T (2005) Research ethics. In: Gerrish K, Lacey E (eds) The Research Process in Nursing. Blackwell, Oxford.

Jones D (1975) Food for thought. Royal College of Nursing, London.

Lawton J (2000) The dying process: Patients' experiences of palliative care. Routledge, London.

London Health Observatory (2005) Prevalence of cardiovascular disease. LHO, London.

Luker K (1984) Reading nursing: the burden of being different. International Journal of Nursing Studies 21(1), 1–7.

Milgram S (1974) Obedience to authority: an experimental view. Harper and Row, New York.

Mitchell M (2001) Constructing information booklets for Day Case patients. International Journal of Ambulatory Surgery 9(1), 37–45.

Moskop JC, Marco CA, Larkin GL, Gelderman JM, Derse AR (2005) From Hippocrates to HIPAA: Privacy and confidentiality in emergency medicine – Part 1: Conceptual, moral and legal foundations. Annals of Emergency Medicine 45(1), 53–59.

Oakley A (1990) Who's afraid of the randomized controlled trial? Some dilemmas of the scienfic method and 'good' research practice. Women and Health 15(4), 25–59.

Pearcey P, Elliott B (2004) Student impressions of clinical nursing. Nurse Education Today 24(5), 382–387.

Seal D, Bloom F, Somlai A (2000) Dilemmas in conducting qualitative sex research in applied field settings. Health Education and Behavior 27(1), 10–23.

Seymour J (2001) Critical moments – death and dying in critical care. Open University Press, Bucks.

The Royal College of Nursing Research Society (2003) Nurses and research ethics. Nurse Researcher 11(1), 7–21.

Warwick D (1973) Tearoom trade: means and ends in social research. Hastings Centre Studies 1, 27–38.

Watson R (1996) Product testing on trial. In: de Raeve L (ed.) Nursing Research: An Ethical and Legal Appraisal. Baillière Tindall, London.

White A, Johnson M (2000) Men's experiences of chest pain: Niggles, doubts and denials. Journal of Clinical Nursing 9, 534–541.

Wiles R, Ashburn A, Payne S, Murphy C (2004) Discharge from physiotherapy following stroke: the management of disappointment. Social Science & Medicine 59(6), 1263–1273.

Williamson TK (2003) Building the evidence base for shared governance: the Rochdale experience. In: Edmonstone J (ed.) Shared governance: making it work. Kingham Press, Chichester.

Williamson TK (2004) Strengthening decision-making within shared governance: an action research study. Unpublished PhD thesis. University of Salford, Salford.

7

Research governance: an international perspective

Michelle Howarth and Rosie Kneafsey

INTRODUCTION

With the launch of the NHS Research & Development Strategy (Department of Health (DH) 1991) came a growing recognition that the content and delivery of care in the NHS needed to be based on reliable, high-quality research. As a result, the volume of research currently being undertaken in collaboration with NHS patients and staff populations has grown steadily over the last 10–15 years. However, to sustain high-quality research and to encourage an evidence-based culture to thrive, it has become clear that sufficient resources, effective infrastructures, systems and processes are needed to underpin it.

Whilst the ethical aspects of research activity have traditionally been regulated by research ethics committees, a number of high-profile examples of research misconduct identified the need for more stringent, transparent mechanisms for monitoring, supporting and organising research activity. At the same time, an important EU Directive relating to research was also published. As a result, a framework for the proper governance of research was introduced by the UK Departments of Health (e.g. DH 2001a). Aptly entitled, the *Research Governance Framework for Health and Social Care* aimed to develop and promote a quality research culture to ensure the correct, appropriate and robust management of NHS research. Contemporary debate indicates that this framework has resulted in remarkable changes in the subsequent conduct and organisation of research.

This chapter will explore the nature of and implications of the research governance framework ('the framework') and the ways in which it seeks to promote and foster a quality research culture. In addition, the relationship between research governance and the recent introduction of the European Directive for the conduct of clinical trials (EU 2001) will be explored. It will also discuss the impact of the framework on researchers, students and their supervisors.

POLITICAL INFLUENCES ON RESEARCH ACTIVITY

The contemporary political agenda has important influences on the conduct of research in the UK. Since the launch of the first NHS Research & Development (R&D) strategy in 1991 (DH 1991), the drive by the UK government to foster a quality research programme and agenda has been relentless. The NHS R&D strategy and subsequent white papers (DH 1994, 1998a, 1998b, 1999a) have each highlighted the need for research programmes to address the most prevalent health-care problems experienced by the population. As a result, the key health priorities outlined in 'Our Healthier Nation' (DH 1998b) (cancer, mental health, cardiovascular disease and stroke) now influence the national R&D agenda and regionally funded research programmes.

To further support and strengthen the relationship between population health needs and research priorities, the Central R&D Committee (CRDC) was introduced in 1998 to advise the NHS on the investment of research funds and setting of research priorities (CRDC 1998a). The white paper 'Research and Development for a First Class Service' (DH 2000) was also published, which placed greater emphasis on the quality and control of research activity within the NHS and social services. Observable variations in the quality and nature of care across the NHS also stimulated the development of a 10-year strategy to support evidence-based practice through the development of national service frameworks and national guidelines. For the first time, research was now inherently linked through policy to care delivery and organisation.

To enable research to meet the new demands of the political agenda the newly developed CRDC commissioned a report into the funding needs of the NHS to support research activity. The report (DH 1999b) recommended radical changes throughout the NHS R&D funding programme. These organisational changes had far-reaching impacts on NHS research. However, it was still suggested that research activity needed to be more closely monitored, particularly in light of highly publicised cases of poor research practice (see Box 7.1): for example, the failure of

Box 7.1 Examples of poor research practices in the UK

Consent processes and research involving babies

A review was undertaken of practices in the North Staffordshire Hospital Paediatric Department because of complaints about the way in which research studies were being conducted. In particular, this related to the routine use of continuous negative extrathoracic pressure in premature babies and infants with bronchiolitis and the use of covert video surveillance to detect a form of child abuse known as 'Munchausen syndrome by proxy'. Although the review found that the research was carried out broadly in line with guidance issued at the time, it concluded that this was too ambiguous; allowing poor practices to occur and go undetected (NHS Executive 2000). Particular problems related to the process of gaining parents' consent. Many parents felt they had received inadequate explanation and choice and were not involved in decision-making. Accusations were also made that consent forms were forged. Some parents also suggested that the ventilator treatment harmed their babies, causing brain damage and death. The review concluded that tighter methods of monitoring research and stronger guidance on good research practices were needed. The need for robust trials to test the efficacy of the ventilator treatment was also emphasised.

Consent to remove and retain organs

In 1999 a panel was appointed to investigate the removal, retention and disposal of human organs and tissues following post-mortem examination at the Royal Liverpool Children's Hospital for the purposes of medical education and research. The investigation found that the Human Tissue Act of 1961 had been breached and that clinicians had failed to obtain parental consent before removing the dead children's organs. The inquiry identified several levels of failure, for example, with the University and Hospital management and monitoring approach, but also laid criticism with particular individuals such as Professor van Veltzen and the coroner. In particular, van Veltzen was found guilty of ordering the unethical and illegal retention of infant and organ body parts for the purposes of research (although the bulk of organs stored were never used), lying to parents, falsifying records, statistics and research applications and failing to meet clinical duties, specifically histological examination during post mortems. A series of recommendations arose from this report for universities, NHS trusts, clinicians, pathologists, coroners, the DH, the Royal Colleges and medical schools (House of Commons 2001).

researchers to gain parents' consent prior to entering babies into research trials (Smith 2000). Examples such as these undermined public trust and confidence in researchers and threatened the future recruitment of participants into important research studies. It was felt that a framework for the proper governance of research was needed.

THE RESEARCH GOVERNANCE FRAMEWORK

The introduction of the framework has been viewed as a means of regaining public confidence in research in health and social care settings. Whilst some criticisms have been levelled at the framework (see Box 9.1), contained within it are a set of specific standards to which close adherence is required and monitored. The framework clarifies responsibilities and accountabilities and relates not only to clinical and non-clinical research undertaken by NHS staff, but also to that undertaken by universities, charities, industry and research councils. The standards have been designed to ensure that research carried out in health and social care settings is of high scientific quality, is ethical and protects the rights of the participants, prevents the occurrence of adverse incidents, and prevents poor performance and misconduct. In many ways, research governance mirrors or fits within clinical governance, which seeks to ensure that patients receive clinically effective, evidence-based and consistently available care (Squires 2001).

The new framework is of direct consequence to a range of groups such as funders, those who host research, those carrying out research, participants in, or managers of health and social care research. For each party involved a range of specific guidance now exists revolving primarily around five key domains. These domains relate to ethics, science, information, health and safety, finance and intellectual property.

Within the framework document, each domain is described and guidance provided about the specific attributes associated with the domains. Local implementation plans (DH 2001b) with key milestones and deadlines were also developed to help organisations to fulfil the requirements of the framework and to enable research ethics committees (RECs) to implement the new changes (DH 2001b).

THE FIVE DOMAINS OF RESEARCH GOVERNANCE
Ethics

The standard for ethics states that the 'dignity, rights, safety and well being of participants must be the primary consideration in any research study' (DH 2005a, p. 11). Data protection, ethics committees, informed consent and confidentiality are, therefore, key concerns. The need to involve service users in research design and to conduct research that respects the diversity of human life are also highlighted. Previously, no monitoring arrangements were in place to ensure adherence to ethical principles. Once a research protocol was approved by the REC, researchers, although obliged to adhere to ethical practices, were not followed up or monitored. The framework attempts to rectify this by strengthening the power of RECs and the relationship between NHS trusts and RECs.

Science

The science domain identifies that the conduct of poor-quality research and unnecessary research duplication is both wasteful and unethical. It emphasises the importance of researchers using existing sources of evidence to support their own work. This is clearly reflected in the new centralised research ethics form provided by COREC (Central Office for Research Ethics Committees), which stipulates the need for all project proposals to take account of relevant literature, retrieved through a process of comprehensive literature searching. This domain also advises that all projects should be subject to an appropriate level of peer review to ensure that studies are well designed and rigorous. Researchers are also encouraged to seek guidance and supervision from experienced researchers.

Special guidance is also provided for research involving human embryos, animals, genetically modified organisms and medicines. In addition, data archiving is discussed and explicit guidance on the storage, retrieval and management of data is included. NHS organisations are now urged to make sure that systems are in place to monitor compliance with these standards.

Information

A plethora of evidence reports the failure to disseminate and implement research findings and addressing this issue has become a pivotal role of the research governance framework. It is recognised that information on research being undertaken and the results of research must be accessible. All research protocols now need to provide a transparent account of the planned dissemination strategy. In addition, NHS trusts must complete quarterly research returns, which are entered onto the National Research Register. This web-based database provides the public with access to ongoing projects and completed research findings (DH 2005b).

Health and safety

Within the domain for health and safety, it is recognised that some research may involve the use of potentially harmful equipment, substances or organisms. Whilst researchers were not obliged to report or disclose health and safety issues prior to the introduction of research governance, detailed consideration must now be given to the ways in which the safety of participants and staff are to be protected. In addition, the introduction of the Medical Devices Agency (MDA), which was later incorporated into the MHPRA (Medicines and Healthcare Products Regulatory Agency) means that research in which new or existing medical devices will be used must be approved by this body to ensure safety for the staff and the patient.

The health and safety standard has had important impacts on external researchers. For example, it is now the case that researchers who are not employed by NHS organisations, but who are conducting research within the NHS or with NHS populations, must adhere to the same duty of care as those employed by an NHS Trust. External researchers must now obtain an honorary contract with the host organisation in order to undertake research. Whilst this process may delay planned data collection activities (Howarth & Kneafsey 2004), it assures NHS organisations of the credibility and ability of the researcher to undertake the research within their organisation. In addition, patient safety is protected through the activities of human resources departments, which may involve the completion of criminal records bureau check and occupational health check.

Finance and intellectual property

The financial probity of an organisation must be assured if research activity is to take place. In order to comply with the laws and rules relating to the use of public funds, it is essential that all research funds are managed appropriately. Partnership working between R&D departments and finance are seen as vital elements to ensure adherence to this standard. As a result, research protocols must clearly outline the research funding source and provide detailed costing and management plans. In addition, compensation for anyone harmed as a result of studies should be made available and indemnity of the researcher assured. This has had implications on those who 'sponsor' research, and indemnify projects. In an attempt to promote the success of sponsorship arrangements, the DH has a recognised list of sponsors. Sponsors are organisations who provide indemnity of the researcher or at least ensure that adequate arrangements are in place. Recent EU Directives (EU 2001) have, however, provoked some reticence about the role, given the implications of failed indemnity.

The domain for intellectual property (IP) is concerned with inventions, knowledge, copyrights and database rights, designs, trademarks and materials, and provides clear guidance about the monitoring and protection of IP within the NHS. This standard seeks to address the previous failure of NHS organisations to capitalise on commercial opportunities and benefits potentially arising from research undertaken within NHS settings. Indeed, many patents, good ideas and potential new technology have previously been exploited by outside agencies and companies.

SUPPORTING THE DEVELOPMENT OF A QUALITY RESEARCH CULTURE

As well as setting standards to ensure best practice in research activity, the framework also describes the key attributes of a quality research culture where 'excellence is promoted and where there is visible and strong research leadership and expert management' (DH 2001a, p.14). The following key principles are seen as essential within a quality research culture:

- Respect for participants' dignity, rights, safety and wellbeing
- Valuing the diversity within society
- Personal and scientific integrity
- Leadership
- Honesty
- Accountability
- Openness
- Clear and supportive management.

The framework advocates that clear agreements and frameworks should be devised that specify the key responsibilities of each party involved in the research activity. These are broadly described within the framework (see Box 7.2) in relation to those organisations undertaking, sponsoring, funding or hosting research. In addition, it is recommended that performance is monitored against responsibilities to ensure that failures to adhere to the standards for best research practice are identified and rectified. Reports of this monitoring are forwarded to the Secretary of State for Health and failing organisations are required to produce recovery plans to improve the governance of research.

In addition to these responsibilities, further requirements are set out within the EU Directives relating to clinical trials (EU

Box 7.2 Roles and responsibilities

- **Researchers:** Responsible for the day-to-day running of the project
- **Principal researcher:** It is essential that a principal investigator (PR) be designated for any research undertaken in the NHS. The PR needs to have sufficient expertise to be able to manage the design, conduct, analysis and reporting of the research
- **Sponsor:** The role of the sponsor is to ensure the quality of the research environment and the competence of the research personnel. The sponsor IS NOT the funder. The sponsor ensures adequate indemnity for the research project and carries a weighty responsibility for the overall conduct of the research
- **Organisational funding:** The organisation that funds the research has a responsibility to support and develop a quality research culture
- **Organisation providing care:** This is the organisation which 'hosts' the research. The host organisation is responsible for ensuring that it has the capacity to host the research and that the patients are not harmed during its conduct. It must also maintain an accurate record of all research activity within the organization.

2001) and which have been incorporated into UK domestic law since April 2004.

EUROPEAN UNION DIRECTIVES

In April 2001, the European Parliament and the Council of the European Union published a directive for the good conduct and monitoring of clinical trials involving human subjects and medicinal products (EU 2001). Whilst the Directive provides guidance on a wide range of issues relating to clinical trials, the key principles outlined relate to the protection of research subjects. Particular attention is given to the protection of vulnerable persons (such as children or those with mental illness) who may not be able to provide legal consent. It is advised that where possible only those persons who are capable of providing consent should be included in trials. However, when there are grounds for assuming a direct benefit that outweighs the risks, vulnerable populations may be included with care if written consent is obtained from the person's legal representative. More recently, additional guidance on good clinical practice (Commission Directive 2005/28/EC) was implemented in January 2006, setting further standards regarding good practice in the design, initiation, conduct, recording and reporting of clinical trials.

In a similar way to the framework, the EU Directive advocates that good monitoring and recording systems are in place for all clinical trials. To monitor this, researchers must provide information, subject data and documents which justify the involvement of human subjects in a trial. The EU Directive also stipulates the need for researchers to ensure that adverse events and reactions are recorded and reported. All information pertaining to the conduct, organisation, management and monitoring of the clinical trial must also be made available for external scrutiny.

The EU Directive was transposed into UK law in May 2004 by the Medicines for Human Use (Clinical Trials) Regulations 2004 (EU 2001). The EU Directive, therefore, is of direct relevance to the research sponsor, the host organisation, the funder and the researcher. Efforts to become familiar with the content and adhere to the Directive should be considered at the outset of any research activity. In an attempt to reduce the ambiguity and promote compliance with both research governance and the EU Directive, the Medical Research Council (MRC) together with the DH, have provided researchers and managers with guidance on implementing the Directive in context with local research governance arrangements. This is published in the Clinical Trials Toolkit, which is available on http://www.ct-toolkit.ac.uk.

IMPLEMENTING THE RESEARCH GOVERNANCE FRAMEWORK

Following the publication of the framework, the DH envisaged full compliance with the framework by April 2004. However, it was also recognised that some organisations might struggle with the new demands now placed on them. To address this, a series of compliance milestones was introduced to support organisations through the implementation process. For example, by March 2003, all NHS organisations needed to ensure staff awareness of research governance; that there were links with clinical governance systems; the monitoring of adverse events and all research projects was evident; all research had a nominated sponsor and research by students was approved. The DH in collaboration with Strategic Health Authorities and the Commission for Health Improvement was responsible for the monitoring of compliance with the framework. Although some organisations have successfully implemented governance, others have struggled due to a shortage of resources, limited infrastructures and lack of engagement with those undertaking research.

Indeed, the DH did not stipulate exactly how research governance should be implemented. Moreover, because the governance of research has been decentralised and is now managed and accounted for at a local level, a wide array of diverse research management and governance systems have developed. As a result, governance requirements and processes may vary from one organisation to another. Researchers are therefore often faced with time consuming and lengthy processes which result in, at best, a delay of research activity and, at worst, may freeze and stifle research innovation and activity (Smith 2000, Jones & Bamford 2004, Howarth & Kneafsey 2004, Kneafsey & Howarth 2005). As a result, some have criticised the framework (see Box 7.3) suggesting that it has potentially destroyed the very thing it was introduced to protect (Jones & Bamford 2004). Indeed, contemporary debate about the processes of research governance in the UK indicates much confusion and frustration about the unwieldy nature of local implementation.

Ongoing debate around this issue led to an exploration of the operation of ethics committees and the problems experienced by researchers when initiating new research. The resultant Warner Report (DH 2005a) identified inconsistencies in relation to REC decisions and proposed nine recommendations. One of these recommended that surveys and other non-research activity that presents no ethical issues for human participants should fall out of the remit of NHS RECs. At present, however, it is advisable to contact the REC chair to discuss whether a study does or does not need to pass through the REC. A list of contact details for each REC can be found on the COREC website at www.corec.org.uk.

Some organisations have implemented research governance with great success, often through careful planning and partnership working. However, it is unclear to what extent research governance is being effectively managed across England, despite development of a guide for the management of research governance within primary care (R&D Forum Toolkit, available at www.rdforum.nhs.uk/toolkit.htm). Previous research has identified the need for ongoing support to implement research management and governance (Shaw et al. 2004) and key attributes enabling organisations to fulfil their R&D functions have been identified (Sarre 2003). However, no nationally coordinated

Box 7.3 Criticism of the research governance framework

- **Bureaucratic and unwieldy:** Researchers argue that processes associated with research governance (RG) are slow and complex, leading to project delays. Differences in implementation across localities also mean that researchers must complete many forms, follow different processes and adhere to a range of varying requirements.
- **Potential deterrent to novice researchers:** The confusing and lengthy processes associated with the framework may act as a deterrent to potential researchers, who perhaps have limited time, support or funding.
- **A quantitative bias:** RECs have traditionally been geared towards quantitative research (e.g. clinical trials) and some argue that RG continues this tradition. Whilst clinical trials are more likely to pose potential harms to participants, qualitative or social research typically poses less, if any harm. It is thus argued that research of this type should not be subjected to the same processes as quantitative research.
- **Loopholes in the framework:** There is confusion about how research, audit and evaluation differ and should be defined. The effect of this is to create loopholes in the RGF. For example, if a project is defined as audit or evaluation, it may avoid the scrutiny of a REC, and potentially important ethical issues may remain unresolved.
- **Concern over the credibility of research ethics committees (RECs):** RECs have been criticised for commenting on methodological rather than ethical issues, for discriminating against qualitative research, and for being medically dominated. The research skills and knowledge of committee members have also been questioned. However, the workload of ethics committees has increased dramatically in recent years, with little extra time and resources to ensure member training and adequate review time for study proposals.
- **Weaknesses of the RG infrastructure:** A lack of dedicated R&D staff in some trusts may limit the effectiveness of the framework, leading it to become a paper exercise rather than a robust system of 'policing.'

evaluation has been undertaken to facilitate this and to streamline and coordinate processes. Research undertaken prior to the implementation of the research governance framework in primary care explored a range of governance models and identified varied partnerships developing according to local circumstances (Scalley & Donaldson 1998). Although this research predicted that future research management and governance partnerships would evolve across wider health organisation boundaries and with increasing co-terminosity, it is not clear to what extent this has been realised.

There is the potential for a symbiotic relationship between clinical and research governance. The supportive clinical governance model adopted by many trusts could help to align research and clinical governance and to smooth processes, enabling a quality research culture to flourish. External partnership working between organisations could promote and strengthen research governance. For instance, examples of partnership working in research in Australia's Co-operative Research Centres (CRC) programme illustrate that good partnership working across organisations can strengthen a research culture and support capability and capacity building. Other countries have also developed good research management systems. It may be that comparing these systems will help identify the strengths and weaknesses of the UK governance framework and help to develop existing frameworks.

INTERNATIONAL PERSPECTIVE

High-profile examples of research misconduct are not unique to the UK, but have also occurred in other countries, such as the USA, Australia and the European countries (see Box 7.4). For example, in the USA the death of a teenager Jesse Gelsinger in a gene-therapy trial resulted in the Office for Human Research Protection suspending a series of research programmes. The later deaths of Hoiyan Wan and Elaine Holden Able (Steinbrook 2002) during research trials also caused public outrage, which played an important part in driving the introduction of tightened approaches to the governance of research in the USA and similar levels of legislation.

In 2001, the US Food and Drug Administration Office (FDA) established the Office for Good Clinical Practice in an attempt to co-ordinate efforts to protect research participants (Steinbrook 2002). The FDA now has responsibility for over 50 000 research active investigators and 1000 commercial sponsors of research. The FDA ensures that all projects are monitored and conducts audits and inspections every year. Other changes include the introduction of a system of accreditation in North America and Canada aimed at providing the public and consumers with confidence about the integrity of the research.

Box 7.4 Examples of research misconduct in other countries

Sweden
The University of Gothenburg in Sweden commenced legal action against two researchers and an administrator for illegally destroying patient data collected over a period of 25 years. The data related to a mental condition known as DAMP (deficits in attention, motor control and perception) and is a widely used diagnostic concept in child medical practice in Sweden. At the time that the data were destroyed, a court order launched by two external researchers to independently examine the data archives had been upheld. The two researchers had suggested that the research results relating to DAMP were scientifically flawed and wanted to examine the raw data themselves. However, the data were destroyed before they had the chance to do this (White 2004).

USA
A 24-year-old healthy volunteer taking part in a study relating to asthma died after inhaling a gas called hexamethonium, as part of the trial. The investigation into how the participant died found that the gas used was 'not for drug use' and that the study information sheet misled participants into believing it was a currently used medication. It also failed to mention any of the potentially dangerous toxic effects of the gas. Participants were not therefore able to give their informed consent. The protocol for dealing with adverse events relating to the study was found to be weak: a previous participant had already developed side-effects from the gas, but these were not acted upon and further participants were recruited. A thorough review of evidence relating to the actions of hexamethonium had not been completed prior to the study and a license had not been sought for its use in this context. The external investigation of this case was critical of the process of review of research protocols at the Institute where the study was conducted (Steinbrook 2002).

In other countries, where deaths and adverse events as a result of research mismanagement have not been publicised, robust systems of research governance have yet to be implemented. However, current debate in Australia, for example, suggests that the reliance on ethics committees may be inadequate as a means of ensuring research quality, and frameworks analogous to the UK and USA systems may be needed (Walsh et al. 2005).

IMPLICATIONS OF THE RESEARCH GOVERNANCE FRAMEWORK FOR RESEARCHERS, SUPERVISORS AND STUDENTS IN THE UK

The changes made within NHS R&D have altered the way in which research is now conducted. All professional groups and those within the social care sector need to be aware of these changes and ensure that their research complies with the requirements of research governance and the EU Directive. Indeed, despite local differences in the way the framework has been implemented, the domains within the framework encourage researchers to scrutinise the scientific merit of the research they have planned, giving careful consideration to the way in which the safe, ethical and transparent conduct of the research will be ensured. Figure 7.1 shows how the domains of the framework reflect aspects of the research process. In the early planning stages of a research study during which the research question is refined,

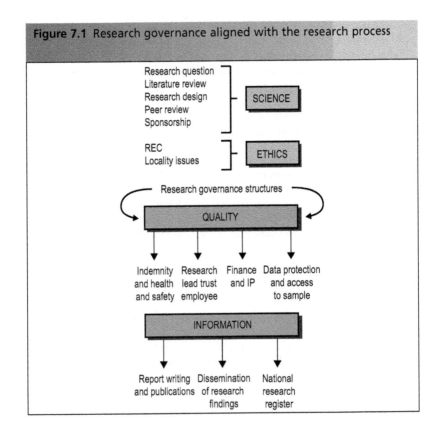

Figure 7.1 Research governance aligned with the research process

the existing evidence base is examined and the design and methodology of the planned study are set out, the science and ethics domain of the framework are especially relevant, ensuring peer review and sponsorship are in place and ethical approval has been gained. By adhering to the requirements of these two domains, the foundations are laid for a study that is able to comply with the rigours of the quality domain. Not only will this ensure the proper conduct of the study and analysis of data, but it will also necessitate that projects are properly managed within the research site. The final domain of the framework draws attention to later phases of the research process, highlighting the importance of disseminating study findings. Although not made explicit, it is also hoped that good-quality research findings are implemented in practice.

In addition, supervisors of research (for example, of masters level and PhD study) need to be familiar with local governance and ethics processes to facilitate the process for their students. This may involve, for example, contacting the local research ethics committee and R&D department to acquire contact details and information about the local research governance arrangements. Most organisations will have now implemented research governance, although there is still evidence of disparity between organisations. However, whilst some processes may differ, the key principles of research governance should be adhered to. In relation to intellectual property and finance, the supervisor is usually indemnified by the university. Again, however, this may differ between organisations and it is the responsibility of the supervisor to check. To adhere to the domain for science, the supervisor must also check the suitability of the methodology selected for clarity and accuracy. If the supervisor is unfamiliar with the research methodology that the student plans to use, it is advisable to link with other researchers who are perhaps more knowledgeable of the particular approach. Linking with a local research investigator based within the NHS organisation may also help to support the student's research study. Generic principles aligned with research governance good practice have been provided to encourage you to question your research (see Box 7.5).

The student must also fulfil certain responsibilities and seek advice from the supervisor about the research protocol, local research governance arrangements and RECs. It is advisable to overestimate the time needed to gain approval and access to sample sites. In some cases, REC approval may not be required.

Box 7.5 Summary guidance for supervisors and research students

- **Ethics:** Identify whether the project requires university, as well as local REC approval. Guidance to determine whether a project is 'service evaluation' can be found on the COREC website. Ensure that the project protocol is adhered to and any changes, if made, are reported to the host organisation and REC.
- **Health and safety:** Identify whether an honorary contract is required. Help student negotiate processes. Contact with MDRA (if medical devices are being tested/used). Ensure familiarity with relevant health and safety policies during the lifetime of the project.
- **Finance and intellectual property (IP):** Ensure an accurate account of funding is provided. IP rights should be discussed and an agreement made. Indemnity arrangements should be checked with the host organisation and the university.
- **Science:** Ensure familiarity and confidence with the methodology being used and subject the protocol to internal and external peer review. Where possible, involve the R&D department within the host NHS organisation. An internally based research investigator may be able to assist with supervision of research in practice.
- **Information:** Ensure that a good dissemination strategy has been planned that takes account of the readability of the written materials likely to be produced and how they will be accessed.

For example, if the project is classified as 'service evaluation', there may be no need to obtain REC approval, although this would need to be discussed with both the supervisor and Chair of the REC. Whatever the outcome, the project will still need to be registered with the organisation's R&D department and must adhere to research governance requirements.

Once approval and registration has been secured, the project protocol must be adhered to. If changes are made, both the supervisor and the research governance representative in the organisation must be informed. This is to ensure that the organisation has an accurate record of the project and is aware of any potential conflicts of interest, risk to research participants and changes to the management of the project. In all cases, where patients are involved in research, the safety of patients is paramount, and guidance and advice must be sought from the organisation's R&D department and the supervisor if any aspects of patient safety are compromised.

CONCLUSION

The face of NHS research has changed since the introduction of the first NHS R&D strategy. Since this time, NHS research has focussed on the health needs of the population and is no longer driven by disparate topics. However, recent controversies signalled the need for the proper governance of research. Not surprisingly, many processes evolved and have since been implemented to combat the possibility of future research adverse events. Whilst some have accused governance of being a bureaucratic juggernaut, others argue that research governance is needed to protect patients. In countries where governance is not in place, a push to implement similar strategies is now becoming apparent.

There is now an overwhelming need to regain public trust in research and to support an evidence-based culture within the NHS. Universally, for evidence-based practice to thrive it is imperative that research governance is promoted at all levels and adhered to. Inevitably, it is beyond the scope of the research governance framework to monitor all research projects and account for all research activity. It therefore rests with all parties involved to ensure good practice to promote the continued conduct of safe, ethical and methodologically sound research practice.

REFERENCES

Commission Directive (2005) Commission Directive 2005/28/EC, Official Journal of the European Union, 91/13-91/19.

www.http://dg3.eudra.org/F2/eudralex/vol-1/DIR_2005_28/DIR_2005_28_EN.pdf, (accessed September 16th 2005)

Department of Health (1991) Research for Health. DH: London.

Department of Health (1994) R&D in the New NHS: Functions and Responsibilities. November 1994. DH: London.

Department of Health (1998a) A First Class Service. Quality in the New NHS. DH. London.

Department of Health (1998b) Saving Lives Our Healthier Nation. DH. London.

Department of Health (1999a) Supporting Research & Development in the NHS (The Culyer Report), September. HMSO: London.

Department of Health (1999b) Strategic Review of the NHS R&D Levy: (The Clarke Report). Central Research & Development Committee of the Department of Health, DH. London.

Department of Health (2000) Research and Development for a First Class Service. R&D Funding in the New NHS. DH. London.

Department of Health (2001a) Research Governance Framework for Health and Social Care. DH. London.

Department of Health (2001b) Research Governance for Health and Social Care. Guidance for Local Implementation Plans. DH. London

Department of Health (2005a) Report of the Adhoc Advisory Group on the Operation of NHS Research Ethics Committees. (Warner Report). DH. London.

Department of Health (2005b) National Research Register. http://www.nrr.nhs.uk/ (Accessed 4th November 2005)

European Parliament (2001) Directive 2001/20/EC of the European Parliament and the Council of the approximation of laws, regulations and administrative procedures of the Member States relating to the implementation of Good Clinical Practice in the conduct of trials on medicinal products for human use, Official Journal of the European Communities' (L121, 01/05/01, pp. 34–44)

House of Commons (2001) Royal Liverpool Children's Inquiry: summary and recommendations, www.rlcinquiry.org.uk, accessed 1st August, 2005

Howarth ML, Kneafsey R (2004) The impact of research governance in healthcare and higher education organisations. Journal of Advanced Nursing 49(6), 675–683.

Jones AM, Bamford B (2004) The other face of research governance. British Medical Journal 329, 280–281.

Kneafsey R, Howarth M (2004) Research governance and the art of defence. Clinical Effectiveness in Nursing 8, 66–67.

NHS Executive (2000) West Midlands Regional Office report of the review into the research framework in North Staffordshire, http://www.doh.gov.uk/pdfs/northstaffsexec.pdf, (accessed 1st August 2005)

Sarre G (2003) Trent Focus. Supporting Research & Development in Primary Care Organisations. Report of the Capacity and Activity in Research Project. Trent Focus Group, http://www.trentfocus.org.uk/Resources/CARPFinalReport.pdf

Scalley G, Donaldson L J (1998) Clinical governance and the drive for quality improvement in the new NHS in England. British Medical Journal 317, 61–65.

Shaw S, Macfarlane F, Greaves C, Carter YH (2004) Developing research management and governance capacity in primary care organisations: transferable learning from a qualitative evaluation of UK pilot sites. Family Practice 21(1), 92–98.

Smith R (2000) Babies and consent: yet another NHS scandal. British Medical Journal 320, 1285–1286.

Squires S (2001) Building a culture of evidence based care. Professional Nurse Supplement 16 (6), S2.

Steinbrook R (2002) Improving protection for research subjects. The New England Journal of Medicine 346(18), 1425–1430.

Walsh MK, McNeil JJ, Breen KJ (2005) Improving the governance of health research. Medical Journal of Australia 182(9), 468–471.

White C (2004) Destruction of data prompts calls for Swedish agency to investigate research misconduct. British Medical Journal 329, 72.

8

Getting ethics approval
Carol Haigh

INTRODUCTION

The management of ethics approval for health and social care research has been affected by developments both in governance procedures at national and international levels and by the increase in research activity by health and social care professionals who at one time would not have seen research as part of their role. The purpose of this chapter is to provide an overview of the evolution and role of research ethics committees (RECs). When and how to apply for ethics committee review will be discussed, and the final element of this chapter will focus upon some of the common-sense approaches available to the applicant that will help to facilitate a smooth passage and positive outcome through any ethics committee process. This will be achieved by exploring common reasons for the refusal of ethical permission and also by emphasising the strategies by which a researcher can ensure a favourable REC decision. Throughout the chapter the UK will be used as a primary exemplar case study. However, many of the principles and strategies outlined within this chapter will be the same for countries other than the UK, as will the potential sources of support.

THE DEVELOPMENT AND ROLE OF ETHICS COMMITTEES IN THE NEW MILLENNIUM

The principal goal of European policies in the field of medical research and clinical trials is the protection of human subjects who participate in those clinical trials (Fuchs 2002). Thus, the aim of ethics committees is to ensure medical and scientific aspects of a research proposal can be reconciled with the welfare of research subjects and broader ethical implications. They are charged with providing independent advice to researchers and protecting the dignity, rights, safety and wellbeing of all actual or potential research participants.

In the UK (and much of the EU follows a similar model), RECs are formed of a voluntary membership, of which one-third are lay members (i.e. non-health-care related) with the rest of the committee members providing medical, educational and scientific experience and expertise. The whole is supported by a local administrator and by the Central Office of Research Ethics Committees (COREC). UK RECs share their role and responsibilities with others as described in the Department of Health's (DH) publication in 2001: *Research Governance Framework of England*. It is important to point out at this stage that, although a consideration of the role of research governance committees is not the remit of this chapter, in the UK no research project can commence until *both* ethics and governance approval have been obtained.

Fuchs (2002) notes that despite the differing historical roots of the various ethics committees and the diversity of ethics review systems in use across Europe the protection of human beings is a universal and fundamental principle. Partly in an effort to address the Europe-wide discrepancies in the management of ethics review of health research and partly to engage in the debate regarding inconsistencies in the supervision of clinical trials, the EU Clinical Trials Directive was drafted. The directive (2001/20/EU) was published in May 2001, became part of UK legislation in 2003, and was fully implemented by 2004. Although the directive's primary focus is upon clinical trials, the standards contained within it are applied to all research proposals that are subjected to ethics review in the UK. This means that:

- Local ethics committees have a maximum of 60 days from receipt of a valid application to give a reasoned opinion
- Ethics committees are allowed one opportunity to seek supplementary information from the applicant. The 60-day time period is suspended until that information is received, then the clock starts ticking again
- With certain exceptions (for example, research concerning gene therapy or somatic cell therapy), the 60-day period cannot be extended.

The main consequences of the EU directive were two-fold. Firstly, the fact that prior to 2001 there had been no regulatory body responsible for the conduct of ethics committees within the UK needed to be addressed. This was achieved by the development of the United Kingdom Ethics Committee Authority (UKECA), which is responsible for outlining the operating areas and working procedures of research ethics committees, accrediting committees to undertake certain kinds of work and which also has the power to abolish committees if necessary.

The second consequence of the directive was that a number of research definitions were articulated to ensure that their meanings could not be misinterpreted. These were outlined in article 2 of the directive and include:

> *Protocol. This is a document that describes the objectives, design methodology and organisation of a study. All REC applications required a protocol to be included as part of the submission*
>
> *Investigator(s). This refers to individuals taking part in a research project as part of the study team. The person who has overall responsibility for the conduct of a study is known as the Chief Investigator. If a study is carried out on more than one site there will be a Principal Investigator at each site who will have responsibility for the study at that site. A site is the place where the research is taking place*
>
> *Site-specific assessment. This assessment is generally carried out for multi-site studies. The assessment is made by members of the relevant local ethics committee who advise the main REC of the suitability of the local investigators and the appropriateness of the local research facilities*
>
> (Central Office for Research Ethics Committees 2004)

Within the UK a strong driver for change and champion of the EU directive was the Pharmaceutical Industry Competitiveness Task Force (PICTF). In its Clinical Research Report (2001) PICTF outlined the need for the development of clinical trials agreements to address not only the standards laid down by directive 2001/20/EU, but also the effects that long drawn out ethics and governance procedures could have upon the start up times of clinical trials. The performance indicators developed within the report, which included reducing the number of trials referred or deferred by ethics committees, reinforced the implementation of the EU directive.

WHEN TO APPLY FOR ETHICS APPROVAL

The requirements of ethics committees are under constant review (DH 2005) and it is not always clear to researchers (especially novice or student researchers) whether their study will require ethics approval. For some students, it is unlikely that their projects will require full consideration by a REC, however, such students should be aware that most, if not all, UK universities have set up their own ethics review committees and such studies will always be reviewed by them. Furthermore, there are strong indications that sooner or later such university research ethic committees (URECs) will be complemented by "triage" mechanisms within COREC outlined by Lilleymunn (2006). All ethics committees, university or NHS, UK or European are serviced by an administrator, and at present, if in any doubt about the requirement for ethics review as applied to specific studies, researchers are encouraged to find out who the administrator is and to seek help and clarification from them. Table 8.1 shows the types of studies for which ethics review will always be required.

From 2004, UK ethics committees also review research studies that are likely to use or access NHS premises and/or use NHS staff as subjects. However, these are two of the issues that are under review (DH 2005). Within the UK there is a considerable

Table 8.1 Studies requiring ethical approval

Study using....	Rationale
Patients and users of the NHS (or any other non-UK health-care system)	This is to protect individuals who may be approached to take part in research projects at a time when they are at their most vulnerable
Relatives/carers of NHS (or any other non-UK health-care system) patients	If relatives and carers are to be approached using NHS databases or recruited on NHS premises then REC approval must be obtained. The case may be different if relative and carers are recruited via organisations external to the NHS – support groups for example. If you are in any doubt consult the REC administrator
Access to data, organs, and other bodily material past and present Access to foetal material Access to the recently dead in NHS premises	In the UK all of theses are governed by the Human Tissue Act 2004 (UK Government). If your research is likely to involve any of these you would be well advised to seek expert advice before continuing with your ethics application

amount of debate regarding the difference between research projects that require ethics committee approval and audit projects that, at the moment, do not, even though audit projects often utilise the same samples and methods as research projects and face the same ethical dilemmas (Johnson 2003). There is guidance on the COREC website regarding the difference between these two activities, but if in any doubt the researcher should seek advice from the relevant REC administrator or from COREC itself before applying to the committee.

The researchers who are the most successful in their ethics committee applications are the ones who include ethical calculations at all stages of their research proposal development. Therefore, before even submitting the documentation for ethics review, potential REC applicants should have:

- Fully developed their proposal
- Explored and agreed the extent of collaboration from other sources (other universities, other sites, etc.)
- Identified the potential sites in which the study will take place
- Obtained (or applied for) university ethics approval if appropriate
- Discussed the project with host research and development office(s)
- Obtained an objective peer review.

When all of these things have been done, the researcher is ready to complete the ethics form and apply for review.

HOW TO APPLY FOR ETHICS REVIEW

Providing it is not a clinical trial of a new medicinal product, a study that is to be held on one site can be considered by the local research ethics committee (LREC). If the study is held on numerous sites that fall within one domain, that is an area that is the remit of one specific body such as a primary care trust (PCT) or an NHS Trust then the application can be reviewed by any local research ethics committee in that area. If a study is being held on two sites that are geographically distinct, i.e. in two domains, and are managed by different trusts the applicant has the option of submitting to both the LRECs that service those areas. For studies that are held on more than two geographically distinct sites, the applicant is best advised to submit to a multi-site research ethics committee (MREC). Submission to an MREC involves ethics review by just one main committee with a decision that is applicable UK wide. The form and supporting materials that are submitted are the same regardless of which of these options the applicant has to choose. The main difference is in the application procedure.

If the study is for consideration by an LREC the applicant can telephone directly to the administrator of their local committee to book in their application. In the UK, details of every LREC administrator can be found via the COREC website (www.corec.org.uk). If the applicant is advised that the next agenda is full, their application can be transferred to another REC. However, this transfer can be declined and the 60 days outlined by the EU directive then begins from the closing date of the next local meeting with an available slot.

All clinical trials with medicinal products, even single site studies, have to go to a recognised REC. In the UK a 'recognised' REC is one that has been approved by the UKECA to review this kind of research study. These trials have to be booked in through a central booking system. Likewise, all other multi-site studies that take place in more than one domain have to go to a 'recognised' REC via this central booking system. In this case the applicant phones COREC when they are ready to submit their study for ethics review, a reference number is assigned to them and a suitable slot in any of the national MRECs is identified. This allocation is confirmed by email and the applicant should ensure that their documentation is forwarded to the MREC within 4 working days. As with the direct application approach for LREC, the MREC applicant can choose not to take the first available slot. If an appropriate slot is declined, the 60 days will start from the closing date of the meeting to which the application is assigned.

THE DECISION-MAKING PROCESS

When an ethics committee meets it considers a number of applications that cover a wide range of health and social care-related research. How the review is managed varies from committee to committee, with some RECs assigning the review of specific applications to certain members of the committee. When this model is adopted the main reviewer is usually the one who will lead the questioning of the applicant with support from the rest of the committee. Other committees expect all members to review all applications and, following some discussion in which the opinions of all the committee members are sought, one member of the committee will lead the questioning with the help of the committee chair. Some researchers can find this process quite daunting but it should be borne in mind that the committee is generally motivated by a desire to contribute to the robustness of the applicant's study by ensuring that the participants and the researcher are fully protected. Student applicants who have submitted to a REC as part of their studies are allowed to take their supervisor to the committee meeting with them as an extra source of support, and this is recommended.

An ethics committee applicant may receive one of three decisions from the committee. The most hoped for option is to obtain a favourable opinion in which the application is approved with no amendments and the study can proceed immediately the written approval is received. The most common decision is a provisional decision in which the committee is minded to approve the study, subject to a number of clarifications or improvements being made to the application or in the supporting material. If the amendments are minimal they are usually submitted to and approved by the chair of the committee, which means that the application does not need to be reviewed again by the full REC and the study is not unnecessarily delayed. If the committee is not convinced that the study is ethically acceptable, or if the application requires major and significant amendments, then the committee will record an unfavourable opinion.

REC applicants do have the right to appeal if they disagree with the decision of the committee. If the appeals process is initiated, the same application will be submitted to a second and different ethics committee. The decision of this second committee is considered as final. Any application that receives an unfavourable decision can be revised and submitted as a new application to the original REC.

WHY IS ETHICS APPROVAL WITHHELD?

Box 8.1 outlines some of the factors that contribute to ethical permission being withheld. These can broadly be placed into one of two categories; methodological robustness and rigour or participant safety.

Methodological robustness

If an ethics committee is not convinced of the robustness and scientific background of a proposed study they are likely to withhold approval. Some committees may give provisional approval subject to a number of queries and conditions being addressed, but this will slow down the progress of any study and is a matter of concern to the researcher. There is a debate in the

---

Box 8.1 Factors that contribute to ethics permission being withheld

- Lack of clear research question
- Vague, unclear or unscientific methodology
- No clear understanding of research philosophies selected
- Lack of statistical advice
- Sample size (too large or too small)
- Lack of peer review
- Non-inclusion of the research tools to be used (questionnaires/interview schedules)
- Lack of consideration for research participants
- Lack of support mechanisms if participants become upset
- Lack of consideration for the researcher
- Lack of supervision for student studies
- Poorly constructed participant- or patient-information sheet

---

UK as to whether ethics committees should concern themselves with the scientific justification and power of research studies with a suggestion that, in the majority of cases, this is outside the remit and expertise of committee members (DH 2005). Conversely, there is a wider international school of opinion that suggests that unscientific research is unethical in nature and that to subject study participants to data collection that is poorly constructed, unlikely to contribute overall to scientific progress or to advance the knowledge of a specific discipline is ethically inappropriate, morally indefensible and, as such, is a key role of the REC (NSW Department of Health 2003, FLACEIS 2003). These arguments notwithstanding, any REC application that does not clearly and explicitly state the research question, the methods by which this question is to be answered and the underpinning philosophies and knowledge base to which the study will contribute is not likely to promote a good impression at the committee stage. Ethics committee members are likely to be impressed or otherwise by the quality of the proposal before them in terms of its clarity of thought and objectives.

In the past, in the UK, the main work of research ethics committees was to evaluate the ethical focus of randomised controlled trials (RCTs) and this historical footprint is still evident in the REC form of today with a significant amount of information being required regarding the statistical rigour of sample size and selection and data analysis. Although it has been recommended that the form is amended to reflect the more qualitative nature of much of health and social care research (DH 2005), at present the form does encourage researchers to give careful consideration to these issues as they impact upon their proposed study. Whilst it is important that qualitative researchers clearly articulate *why* statistical advice may be inappropriate for their study, it is equally important that quantitative researchers clearly show the planning and rationale that is underpinning their proposed study and how quantitative data analysis selected will contribute to robust results that have statistical and/or clinical meaning. Additionally, some RECs may have difficulty understanding the necessarily small sample sizes that are often attendant upon qualitative research and qualitatively focussed applicants should be prepared to explain and defend their small sample sizes with as much vigour as quantitative researchers should when defending their larger sample sizes. Furthermore, many RECs would find it easier to give approval to proposed studies if data-collection tools, such as questionnaires and interview schedules were submitted as part of the application. Not only would this facilitate the committees in their work in protecting the public, it would allow for an informed evaluation to be made of the analytical techniques proposed by the applicant. It can be very frustrating for a researcher to find that their ethics approval has been held up pending the provision of a simple data-collection tool that should have formed part of the primary application; however, RECs would argue that if they do not have sufficient information to evaluate the public risk inherent in the proposal, they have an obligation to suspend or withhold consent.

Many of the problems that can face research ethics committee applicants could be addressed by a stringent system of peer review prior to, and included in, submission to the REC. Surprisingly, peer review as part of the ethics process is not widely utilised in many countries that are operating formal research ethics approval processes (Institute of Science & Ethics 2002). In the USA, peer review was seen as pre-dating the formal REC system and in Europe peer review is not even mentioned in the 'Guidelines and recommendations for European Ethics Committees' document (European Forum for Good Clinical Practice 1997). Even in countries that do operate such a system, it is often informal and is a subjective 'friend' or 'colleague' rather than an objective 'peer' review and, furthermore, is sporadic in application. In the UK there is a suggestion that a rigorous system of national expert peer review panels be set up to ensure that the scientific rigour and appropriateness of studies are considered before submission to RECs (DH 2005), and this would go a long way to improving the quality of submissions to and the approval rate of RECs .

Participant safety

This focuses upon the safety of the research respondents and upon the researchers themselves, all of whom can be argued to be participants in the entire research process. Therefore, if a lack of consideration for the wellbeing of the participants is evidenced by omissions or actions, such as under- or overestimating potential participant vulnerability, underrating the possibility of distress being caused by certain interview topics or disregarding a potential need of outside support for respondents as a result of issues raised in the research study, then ethics committees will withhold approval until these issues are addressed to their full satisfaction.

The importance of informed consent is fully emphasised by most REC documentation throughout Europe, and the UK is no exception (Fuchs 2002). However, there is more to informed consent than providing a suitable consent form, and a number of research ethics applications are turned down due to overly jargonised or downright incomprehensible patient-information sheets. The information sheet should be designed to communicate clearly to potential study participants the nature of the research, the role that they will be asked to play within it and how they are to be protected whilst they participate. There is an art to producing a good information sheet that a surprising number of researchers (not all of them novices) do not have. If an ethics committee has any concerns that the information given to potential recruits is misleading or incomplete it will withhold its approval.

Two main issues arise when the safety of the researcher is considered. The first one is of primary concern in health and social care research that is taking an ethnographic or phenomenological approach and is seeking information from participants in their own environment; for example, observing how parents interact with their children in the home or interviewing or observing individuals in environments not of the researcher's choosing. Such scenarios provide RECs with concerns regarding security of the researcher. The development of an inclusive risk governance culture is a key part of European Union activities in the field of science and society (European Commission 2005) and UK universities are working to develop their own lone-worker policies within the guidelines of the UK Health and Safety Executive

(2005). An example of a good lone-worker practice can be found at the website of the Office of Research and Enterprise of Keele University.[1]

Although it can be argued that such concerns are more usually addressed by research governance rather than by RECs, researchers would be well advised to seek out information regarding such policies prior to submitting their ethics approval application if they do not want a delay in obtaining approval. If such a policy is not in existence, the development of a simple 'buddy' system whereby the lone researcher arranges a contact time with a colleague is often sufficient to satisfy an ethics committee.

The second of the protection and safety issues that exercise ethics committees is that of sufficient and suitable supervision for student research. In the UK it has been suggested that ethics committees focussed specifically upon the research work carried out by students at all levels of education up to and including master level should be created, with PhD work being seen as research rather than education and reviewed by RECs (Doyal 2004). Underpinning this is the need for supervisors of students to be aware of the proposed activities of the student researchers and to be able and willing to provide support, guidance and advice throughout the life of project, including the ethics approval stage. RECs will and do withhold their approval if they do not feel that there is sufficient emphasis on supervision within a student proposal. The argument, again, is that novice research must be under the direction of an experienced researcher if the interests of the student and the public are to be safeguarded.

Thus, it can be seen that a number of factors, either singularly or cumulatively, can contribute to ethics approval being withheld by a research ethics committee. However, it must be stressed that the researcher has the power to address the majority of them and should have given them all due consideration before even applying for ethics approval. Since the obtaining of ethics approval is one of the fundamental steps on the research pathway, a sensible and competent researcher will ensure that their application is as accurate as it can be prior to submission. To this end the next segment of this chapter will explore some of the strategies available to a researcher to ensure that their application is received favourably by the REC.

---

[1] http://www.keele.ac.uk/research/researchgovernance/loneworking.htm#top

HOW TO IMPROVE A RESEARCH ETHICS COMMITTEE SUBMISSION

One of the most important things a researcher can do when embarking upon an ethics application is to visit the COREC website and read the guidelines for applicants. These guidelines, in conjunction with the Frequently Asked Questions page of the site will go a long way to helping with completion of the ethics form, which can look quite daunting to novice researchers. The principles contained within these guidelines can also help if completing ethics forms for review outside of the UK in the case of international research.

Many of the factors that help to make a REC application successful can be described as 'application linked'. This relates to the common-sense approaches that involve the presentation of information. RECs review, on average, eight to 10 applications per month and, although the committee tries to be objective, it will draw its own conclusion about the academic and scientific skills of the researcher if the application is badly completed. Simple strategies such as intense proof reading and spell checking of the document prior to submission can considerably enhance the chance of approval.

Another important thing to bear in mind is the fact that ethics applications are read and approved by people who may not be completely familiar with many areas of expertise, so it is crucial that jargon and abbreviations are avoided. It is also important that the injunction laid upon applicants to provide their information 'in language a lay person can understand' is adhered to. If an applicant has tried hard to communicate their ideas clearly and simply, an ethics committee is likely to view their application favourably. This clarity of communication can be achieved if a significant amount of thought has gone into the project prior to commencing the ethics approval application and if the researcher has considered how the aims and objectives of their proposed study relate to their stated research question. In the UK the average reading age of the adult population is that of an educated 9 year old, comparing poorly with EU countries such as Sweden and The Netherlands. This should be seen as a guide when producing information literature, etc.

There are two pitfalls that beset researchers completing the research ethics application form. One is the desire to provide as much detail as possible to the REC. This can work against an applicant since providing more information than is requested can lead ethics committees into areas of inquiry that may be unprofitable to the researcher. For example, if a researcher has identified that there is a small possibility of distress being caused by their questions at interview, it should be sufficient to reassure the REC that appropriate measures are in place to support such an event and to outline briefly what those measures may be. If the researcher gets too deep into a discussion of how unlikely such distress may be the committee may become entrenched in the debate rather than approving the arrangements that have been made. So answers should be carefully considered, and an applicant should provide solely the detail asked for and not elaborate. If a REC wants more information it will ask for it.

If one of the pitfalls is the provision of too much information, the other occurs when the applicant does not provide sufficient detail for the committee to base a judgement upon. Thus, it is important that the applicant answer every question on the form. If a question is not applicable to the study under consideration, the applicant must say so and state why. Only authors of complex (and highly unlikely) multi-site studies of new drugs on prisoners who are pregnant and have mental-health problems, with the use of additional radiation and using stored blood samples are ever likely to have to complete the form in its entirety. However, if a question is left unanswered the ethics committee does not know whether it is because the question is inapplicable to the study or whether it is an error or oversight on the part of the applicant. Approval may be deferred while this deficit is remedied.

The application forms for RECs in the UK can appear over-whelmingly complex to the uninitiated. Nonetheless, however comprehensive they appear, the forms rarely provide RECs with all of the information that they need in order to review the proposed study thoroughly. Therefore, a REC application should comprise any number of supporting documents including, at least, patient-information leaflets, research protocols, a consent form, letters to GPs (possibly), a questionnaire, interview schedules and recruitment posters. Many RECs invite applicants along to meetings to explain their study and to answer questions from the panel and this is an opportunity that a researcher should be quick to accept. Actually being at the ethics committee meeting to defend an application does help to address any potential problems and can speed up approval for the study. Box 8.2 summarises the actions that researchers can take that will strengthen their submission to the research ethics committee.

Some ethics committees will allow individuals to attend their meetings as an observer; this can be an interesting and

---

Box 8.2 Factors that contribute to ethics permission being conferred

- Read the guidance notes
- Complete every question
- Don't answer 'none' to any question relating to major ethics issues – there has to be something – that's why the proposal is submitted
- Think carefully about all answers
- If the ethics form says 'in language a lay person can understand' it really means it
- Avoid abbreviations and jargon
- Answer only what the question asks
- Give details of literature searches
- Be extremely clear what exactly the study is trying to achieve
- Give careful thought to recruitment methods
- Proof read everything
- Provide information about data collection tools: questionnaire, interview schedules, etc.

---

educational experience and can give potential applicants insight into how the entire ethics review process operates. The appropriate REC administrator will be able to provide information about the feasibility of such visits.

CONCLUSION

Within Europe the basic standards of ethics committee reviews are articulated by the EU directive 2001/20/EU (European Commission 2001). Although the directive is primarily concerned with the management of clinical trials involving new medicinal products, in the UK the directive has been taken as the standard for the review of all projects that involves NHS patients, premises or staff.

There are a number of strategies that a researcher can implement in order to ensure a positive decision from any review committee, be it local or multi-site. Most of these involve full and comprehensive review of all the potential ethical dilemmas inherent in a study at the planning stage to ensure that the application is as informative as it needs to be. Furthermore, constant proof reading and careful construction of all patient and lay person information materials will go some way to facilitating the desired outcome. Finally, ethics review committees take their role of protectors of the public extremely seriously and an implied part of that role includes protecting the academic reputation of the researchers themselves. So, although it can be frustrating for a REC applicant to find that they have to review certain aspects of their proposed study or provide the committee with extra information or materials, it should also be remembered that such demands are in the best interest of the study participants and the researcher themselves.

REFERENCES

Central Office for Research Ethics Committees (2004) New Operational Procedures for NHS RECs. Available at http://www.corec.org.uk/recs/guidance/docs/Guidance_for_Applicants_to_RECs.pdf (accessed 20.06.05)

Department of Health (2005) Report of the ad hoc advisory group on the operation of NHS research ethics committees. London: DH

Doyal L (2004) The Ethical Governance and Regulation of Student Projects: A Draft Proposal. Available at www.corec.org.uk/recs/docs/SPECs_proposal_DRAFT.doc (accessed 19.06.05)

European Commission (2001) Directive 2001/20/EU. Good Clinical Practice on the conduct of clinical trials. Available at http://www.corec.org.uk (accessed 20.06.05)

European Commission (2005) Scientific Advice and Governance. Overview of activities. Brussels: European Commission.

European Forum for Good Clinical Practice (1997) Guidelines and recommendations for European Ethics Committees. Brussels: EFGCP.

FLACEIS (Foro Latinoamericano para Miembros de Comités de Ética en Investigación en Salud) (2003) Guidelines followed by a research ethics committee. http://www.flaceis.org/flaceisinfo.php?cat=01010200&i=1 (accessed 19.06.05)

Fuchs M (2002) Final draft report : Provision for support for producing a European directory of Local Ethics Committees (LECs). Institute of Science and Ethics, University of Bonn, Germany.

Health and Safety Executive (2005) Working alone in Safety. Controlling the risks of solitary work. HSE. London

Johnson M (2003) Research ethics and education: A consequentialist view. Nurse Education Today 23, 165–167.

Lilleymunn J (2006). Implementing the recommendations of the ad hoc advisory group: consultation. NPSA, London.

NSW Department of Health (2003) Health Ethics. http://www.health.nsw.gov.au/pubs/h/pdf/health_ethics_0903.pdf (accessed 19.06.05)

Pharmaceutical Industry Competitiveness Task Force (2001) Clinical Research Report. London: DH. Available at; http://www.advisorybodies.doh.gov.uk/pictf/pictfclinicalresearch.pdf (accessed 19.06.05)

9

Ethics approval, ethical research and delusions of efficacy

Debbie Fallon and Tony Long

ETHICS APPROVAL AND DELUSIONS OF EFFICACY

In this chapter we chart the development of the UK regulatory processes in health-care ethics including the development of research ethics committees and centralised control in the form of Central Office for Research Ethics Committees (COREC). We argue that whilst the increase in regulation was perhaps a reasonable reaction to the problems faced by the health research community, and is undoubtedly an improvement on previously limited scrutiny, it is a route that is somehow racing towards an approach of bureaucratic standardisation.

We discuss the problems faced by ethics committees in this process together with their attempts to solve them and conclude that what has resulted from this is an over emphasis on ethics *approval* rather than review. We conclude that this regulatory model is now viewed by many as nothing more than a bureaucratic hurdle to be faced not only in terms of access, but also in terms of the gate-keeping of publication opportunities.

A consideration of the current system of research ethics committees (RECs) and research governance for research in health and social care reveals a somewhat distorted relationship between what is thought to be ethical and what is approved that is being overlooked. From this we conclude that RECs are not a necessary or sufficient means of ensuring ethical conduct and question the wisdom of promoting the idea that this is the sole means of approaching research in health and social care.

We consider how the drive towards regulation and attempts at standardisation in health have come to contrast sharply with the approach of self-regulating disciplines in social science: a situation which has raised concerns in some health quarters about 'disparity'. Requests for a single overarching code or guideline (particularly in terms of researching with children) indicate that for those who work within the limits of the RECs, self-regulation appears to be viewed with some suspicion. We suggest that, contrary to this, the social science approach should be viewed as an equally rigorous and effective alternative for research that is not subject to REC review.

We take this point further, suggesting that the current system in health, with its emphasis on the role of the committee over and above that of the researcher, could be detrimental to the health- and social-care research community as a whole, and suggest that one of the fundamental principles of the social-science approach (self-regulation) should not be disregarded by researchers in health. Whilst acknowledging that no amount of regulation will prevent a research maverick, we outline why the current emphasis on achieving ethics approval appeals to the authority of a committee to rubber stamp a gold standard research proposal rather than discussion of ethical dilemmas with peers and colleagues in the research community. We argue that this could be detrimental to the development of researcher skills. The current approach places emphasis on training the regulators, diverting the development of skills in ethical self-regulation through promotion of a bureaucratic approval process that discourages discussion about difficult ethical issues.

The rise of research ethics committees and two decades of disparity

The emergence and subsequent development of RECs and the wider system of central control of research in the UK have resulted from reaction to widely publicised scandalous behaviour by a number of (usually medical) researchers and, more latterly, from repeated attempts to iron out a series of problems that have arisen from these developments (see Box 9.1). It has taken more than three decades to reach the pinnacle of centralised control in the form of COREC and research governance.

In 1967 Pappworth published 'Human Guinea Pigs' in which numerous examples of unethical medical research studies with human subjects in the UK and the USA were detailed (Pappworth 1967). Together with later examples of equally unacceptable conduct, this stimulated the Royal College of Physicians in 1973 to call for the establishment of ethics committees to scrutinise research proposals. The Department of Health and Social Security issued an advisory document on the issues 2 years later. This delay of 8 years typifies the delay between the discovery of untoward events or inadequacies in the system and the institution by

---

Box 9.1 Brief examples of scandalous research behaviour

1965: Hyman V The Jewish Chronic Disease Hospital
In this study, brought to light by Pappworth in 1967, live cancer cells were injected into aged, senile patients to study rejection responses. No consent was sought, and deceitful means were employed to ensure continued participation.

1973: The Tuskegee Syphilis Study
For 40 years the public health service in Tuskegee, Alabama conducted a study of two groups of black male subjects, one group with untreated syphilis, to investigate the course of the disease. No treatment was provided and active steps were taken to ensure that treatment remained unavailable.

2001: The Royal Liverpool Children's Inquiry
It was found that a huge collection of organs from child patients at the hospital had been amassed over decades without procedures to gain consent from parents. One of the aims of the collection was to provide material for research purposes (detailed in Chapter 7).

---

governments of measures to address the problem. Of course, the possibility of effective, competent science being undertaken in grossly unethical research studies had been known about at least since the end of the World War II with the trial of Nazi war criminals including, notably, Luftwaffe scientists undertaking lethal studies on Jews and other political prisoners. The issues were hardly new.

Findings from a survey by the Institute of Medical Ethics (IME) in 1983 (Nicholson 1986) demonstrated the chaotic state of RECs at the time (see Box 9.2). Gross differences were to be seen in nature, operation and perceived purpose between committees. Some of the results indicate obvious ineffectiveness; membership varying between a meaningless 'committee' of 1 person and a hopelessly large membership of 73. As usual, there was no immediate response, and no obvious improvement was to be seen for another decade.

The drive for standardisation

From February 1992 (10 years later) new recommendations from the Department of Health set local research ethics committees (LRECs) on a new footing, with a formal requirement for every

> **Box 9.2** Institute of Medical Ethics Findings 1982–83
>
> - 254 research ethics committees contacted
> - 174 (69%) returned the questionnaire
> - Eight refused to co-operate (name of chair withheld in one case)
> - 153 stated that they expected to review all proposals
> - 21 replied that it was not compulsory for proposals to be submitted. Only seven provided guidelines
> - Membership varied from one to 73 members
> - 49 had 10 or more members
> - 14 had only doctors and nurses on the committee
> - Nine of these had no nurse currently
> - 93 had only one lay member
> - One committee had seven lay members
> - RECs unclear about their task

district health authority to establish and operate a LREC (Department of Health 1991). Yet there was no formal co-operation between LRECs, which acted independently of each other. Major differences could be seen in the operation of neighbouring committees. Middle et al., for example, in an attempt to undertake a survey in England and Wales of children born in 1988, identified 162 LRECs, sent 1116 application forms (118 different formats and up to 10 copies per committee), and estimated the cost of the exercise at £4606. The committees varied greatly in their responses and some took an inordinate length of time to deal with the application (Middle et al. 1995). The problem has not been restricted to the UK. Jamrozik reports on similar difficulties in Australia, for example, and offers the example of the need in large (perhaps international) epidemiological studies for uniformity in data collection and so on; a requirement confounded by many and varied requests from LRECs for local alterations to the protocol (Jamrozik 2000).

The relentless drive to improve the system and to further standardise processes and centralise control led in 1997 to the establishment of the Central Office for Research Ethics Committees (COREC). COREC was set up to manage, advise and monitor the entire system of RECs in the UK, including the new multi-centre research ethics committees (MRECs). Some aspects have certainly changed for the better; notably the introduction of a standard application form to be used by all

RECs, training for committee members, and continual review of the effect of implementation. Other developments have been met with more qualified approval. The standard format for information sheets and consent forms (together with detailed guidance for applicants) must be received with relief by many researchers. Yet for others this standardisation runs contrary to their efforts to respond specifically to their participants' needs and to adopt modes of communication that are more meaningful and 'user-friendly' to them; particularly, for example, when the participants are children. In a social research context, Coomber (2002) illustrates clearly why the requirement for the completion of signed consent forms is simply counter-productive to the desire to protect participants in the case of research with criminal populations. For a while there were signs of likely moderation of control in some dimensions of research. Proposals were put forward for alternative arrangements for students undertaking research, but these have now been shelved.[1] Many problems seem to remain, however.

Muddled purposes and square pegs for round holes

One survey of UK LRECs (Osborn & Fulford 2003) found that most committees experienced some difficulty with applications for research in psychiatric settings, either relating to issues of consent and confidentiality with such participants or concerning the instruments to be used. This is, of course, to be expected, since expertise in every medical specialty client population or social group cannot be available to every committee. The widening scope of research methods in use in social science research or in research with children, for example, will also continue to challenge the expertise of REC members. While many nurse researchers make life unnecessarily difficult by regaling RECs with claims to 'a Heideggerian hermeneutic phenomenological approach' (see Johnson 1999) rather than stating clearly what is planned to be done in a proposed study, there has been a long-standing complaint that RECs are commonly reluctant to accept qualitative research as being equally rigorous or worthwhile as traditional scientific designs (Dolan 1999, Coomber 2002).

Although it was part of the 1992 guidance that LRECs should require that the scientific merit of a proposal had been properly assessed, there has been concern for many years that RECs should

---

[1] http://www.corec.org.uk/applicants/#040127a

restrict their review to ethical issues, leaving methodological matters aside (to be reviewed elsewhere before submission to the REC). This view has finally been accepted by the Department of Health and COREC, and expressed in the Warner Report recommendations.

> *RECs should not reach decisions based on scientific review. In the unusual situation of a REC having reservations about the quality of the science proposed, they should be able to refer to COREC for scientific guidance.*
>
> (Department of Health 2005)

Moreover, the report also acknowledges that some research designs present so little (if any) risk to participants as to be inappropriate for ethics review by a REC.

> *The remit of NHS RECs should not include surveys or other non research activity if they present no material ethical issues for human participants. COREC should develop guidelines to aid researchers and committees in deciding what is appropriate or inappropriate for submission to RECs.*
>
> (Department of Health 2005)

Another problem in relation to methodological issues is that, although the standard COREC application form has been repeatedly revised in response to feedback, it remains focussed primarily upon medical experimentation through clinical trials, with many redundant or meaningless questions for those proposing alternative approaches. Moreover, it is difficult to address the issues that social scientists or other qualitative researchers may wish to bring to the attention of the committee, and there have been calls for alternative versions of the application form (Oddens & De Wied 1995, Kaur & Taylor 1996).

Despite the efforts of COREC to provide adequate training for REC members and to foster a homogenous response across committees, there is no common standard of scrutiny or what should be considered acceptable or otherwise. There is still evidence of wide variance in response to applications, particularly when application is made to LRECs following approval by MREC (Stone & Blogg 1997, Lux et al. 2000, Lewis et al. 2001). Lux et al. conclude that 'the two-tier system of ethical review retains the inefficiencies of the former system' (p.1183). Some RECs are known to be more difficult to 'get through' than others. Even the DH review of RECs (The Warner Report) accepted of RECs that 'there is bound to be a subjective element in ethical opinions.

This makes some variation inevitable, but the extent of inconsistency is clearly an irritation' (Department of Health 2005).

Research governance: a second wave of disparity

Linked to the development of COREC and as a direct result of the Royal Liverpool Children's Hospital (RLCH) organ retention scandal was the creation of the research governance framework (Department of Health 2001) discussed in detail in Chapter 7. It is notable that the system of RECs under COREC had been in existence some years before the discovery of the unacceptable practices at RLCH, and RECs had been in place for decades before without preventing the practices at issue. In fairness, research governance is intended to continue the monitoring of research following approval by one or more RECs and it was this scrutiny that was absent previously. However, while such measures are intended to facilitate rather than to prevent the conduct of sound research, there is evidence that this is simply not the case in practice. For some, research governance seems to have dealt a death blow to large-scale survey research. Exactly the same difficulties encountered in gaining ethics approval from numerous RECs for survey research have been repeated with a vengeance in research governance. Although a unified online application form for research governance has been devised by the NHS R&D Forum,[2] its use is not compulsory in NHS organisations, and it has already been seen that the use of a standardised application form has not prevented continued divergence in decision-making by RECs.

A joint statement by the Community Practitioners' and Health Visitors' Association, the Royal College of Midwives, and the Royal College of Nursing (Community Practitioners' and Health Visitors' Association et al. 2005) expresses the concerns admirably[3] (see Box 9.3).

The bureaucratic juggernaut

So the response in health (and latterly social care) has been to pursue the REC approach relentlessly (together, now, with research governance), continually attempting to fix the problems and make the system work. In some aspects of research the COREC approach has proved to be reasonably effective; notably for some

---

[2] https://www.rdform.org.uk/
[3] http://www.man.ac.uk/rcn/rs/RCMRCNCPHVFeb05.htm

Box 9.3 Extract of the position paper on the implementation of research governance procedures (CPHVA, RCM and RCN 2005)

Together with the appropriate mechanisms for securing funding and university/local research ethics committee approval, researchers now have to face many more levels of scrutiny, each of which may take several months to complete, such as:

- Approval of appropriate user groups
- NHS local research management committee approval
- Seek NHS Honorary Contract
- Criminal Records Bureau Enquiry
- Data protection approval from NHS Trusts
- The intellectual property rights requirements of different organisations

Research in the health services is done primarily to improve patient services and quality of care. It is done secondarily, but importantly, to train health service staff in the collection and interpretation of evidence so that this evidence can finally be made integral to that care. Research governance arrangements, which are often additional to and different from ethical approval, seem to be having the opposite effect. For example:

- There is evidence that both senior and junior researchers are avoiding research in the NHS.
- Even those with honorary NHS teaching contracts are being forced to seek new contracts and other research management arrangements to conduct research, and sometimes in several organisations.
- Even where genuine research risks were low in conducting studies (for example, a small-scale survey of NHS staff on a 'non-sensitive' topic) students have to be given extensions to deal with several levels of external evaluation.
- In order to avoid lengthy scrutiny there is common re-negotiation of projects under new labels, such as audit or evaluation of services (even though the actual ethical issues, if any, remain the same).
- Researchers are getting very different decisions from each of the bodies responsible for approval in a given case.
- It is clear that approval often depends on factors other than the design and main ethical issues in a study.
- Some studies are inappropriately rejected by reason of a design with which a panel may be unfamiliar.
- Approval paperwork encourages researchers to undertake 'convenient' research rather than answer important research questions.

Box 9.3 Extract of the position paper on the implementation of research governance procedures (CPHVA, RCM and RCN 2005) (*Cont'd*)

- The Health Departments and their officials are sometimes inconsistent in the use of research governance procedures.
- Research into a wide range of clinical need is being stifled.
- Instead of reducing the costs of research, it is very likely that these new arrangements greatly inflate the cost of even simple studies to a prohibitive level.

---

traditional scientific methods in clinical research in the NHS. Of course, none of the examples of unacceptable research provided in Box 9.1 above fell into this category, though more recent examples certainly have done so (Pickworth 2000).

It is difficult to establish whether the continued drive to standardisation is a cause or consequence of the difficulties faced by ethics committees. Either way, the result seems to be that RECs are cautiously following the letter rather than the spirit of regulation. This means that even for health researchers who have had more time to become familiar with the multiple layers of scrutiny and bureaucracy (REC, research governance, Caldicott Guardian clearance, and the Data Protection Act 1998) the process of gaining approval before and during a study has become a juggernaut (Tod et al. 2002).

The practical consequences

These overwhelming bureaucratic difficulties could produce damaging consequences at practice level. For example, they prompt some researchers to shun the NHS as a setting for research, to avoid worthwhile topics as being impossible to research effectively in the current climate, or in some cases to 'rebrand' research as audit in order to circumvent the bureaucracy. They have also discouraged students on academic programmes from undertaking data-collection activity as part of their programmes since opportunities for this within the NHS have been greatly reduced. In the interests of a timely completion of their programmes, many students may take dissertation options that do not include data collection, therefore obviating the need to 'get through' ethics. So where previous nurse researchers would have begun their career with research projects that included data collection at both first degree and master's level, it is possible that they may now embark on their first piece of data collection and therefore the practicalities of research ethics, at doctorate level. This must surely have a detrimental impact on the opportunities for the development of ethical researchers. At the dissemination end of the process, the consequences for researchers in health who have undertaken research that has not met the criterion of scrutiny by an ethics committee are much more serious. A brief glance at the author guidelines for an increasing number of scholarly journals will reveal that ethics approval details are a prerequisite for publication. The potential for the waste of valuable research here is great, and unacceptable for research teams, funding bodies and the participants. As we argue throughout, ticking the 'ethics approval' box is only one way of improving the moral relevance of research to the community it serves. Journals and other gatekeepers should require that appropriate ethical issues, and the investigators' approaches to them, are properly discussed, rather than mere repetition of the mantra that this or that committee gave approval.

FROM ETHICS APPROVAL TO ETHICAL RESEARCH: AN ALTERNATIVE APPROACH TO ETHICS REVIEW

In summary, whilst the current situation may be an improvement on previous circumstances, it is still problematic in terms of bureaucracy, diverse expertise amongst committee membership, varied responses and response rates, and disagreement about which proposals should be scrutinised. These issues in turn have seen further attempts at standardisation with the apparent aim of meeting the needs of all interested parties; heading towards a kind of 'one size fits all' process but which crucially still appeals to the authority of the ethics committee to 'approve' it.

We aim here to explore the possible implications of this approach, discussing the issues in the wider research context. We take as a starting point that a great deal of research in health and social care is not eligible for scrutiny by NHS RECs: studies in hospices, voluntary organisations, support groups, charitable organisations and the private sector, for example. Although researchers in these fields will normally be just as concerned with the maintenance of ethical conduct as any other researcher, inevitably there is some disquiet about the possibility of disparities and inconsistencies in the research community, particularly when the participants are considered to be a vulnerable population such as children.

The tradition of self-regulation in the social science disciplines throws the increasingly rigid regulatory processes in health-care research even further into sharp relief, and serious issues are raised for health researchers who may find that they are negotiating the bureaucratic juggernaut when researchers from other disciplines are not. If the current trajectory were followed, then the logical next step would be a call from health researchers for all self-regulating disciplines to adhere to the same strict research processes that they follow regardless of their own disciplinary guidance.

Is this the way forward? Whilst we may not come to any agreement about which approach (whose ethics) is best, what we can do here is consider how the current approach to ethics approval in health might *not* be the answer. We will argue that, although RECs may operate fairly well in terms of scrutinising the calibre of the written proposal document and the initial intent of the researcher, they do not necessarily guarantee ethical research conduct. Furthermore, several indicators suggest that placing too much faith in RECs as a panacea for all problems associated with unethical research may be inadvisable. These issues can be addressed through engaging with two questions: 'Is research that has not been approved, unethical (if not, why can't it be published)?' and 'Is research that has been approved necessarily ethical?'

Ethical research in the social sciences

Alternative approaches have been relied upon for years in other disciplines, demonstrating that RECs are not the only way to guide ethical research. Research in social science has a tradition of self-regulation within professional guidelines. The British Psychological Society (British Psychological Society 2004) and the British Sociological Association (British Sociological Association 2002) maintain standing guidance to members in the form of principles, guidelines, and codes of conduct.

The BSA guidance, which amounts to 61 statements of how members of the association should behave in research activity, includes issues of professional integrity, relationships with participants, funders and sponsors; as well as specific matters relating to consent, confidentiality, covert research, disposal of data, and the rights of participants. Importantly, it also addresses issues of personal integrity and responsibility, as well as the communal responsibility to enhance ethical behaviour among members of the association:

> *The purpose of the statement is to make members aware of the ethical issues that may arise throughout the research process and to encourage them to take responsibility for their own*

ethical practice. The Association encourages members to use the Statement to help educate themselves and their colleagues to behave ethically... The statement does not, therefore, provide a set of recipes for resolving ethical choices or dilemmas, but recognises that it will be necessary to make such choices on the basis of principles and values, and the (often conflicting) interests of those involved. Departures from the principles should be the result of deliberation and not ignorance.

(BSA 2002)

The BPS guidance (similar in many ways) also provides specific guidance to researchers in psychology on issues of, for example, consent, covert research, protection of participants, debriefing and intervention. It concludes with a statement of the responsibility of researchers to indulge in mutual monitoring of compliance with expectations of ethical research:

Investigators share responsibility for the ethical treatment of research participants with their collaborators, assistants, students and employees. A psychologist who believes that another psychologist or investigator may be conducting research that is not in accordance with the principles above should encourage that investigator to re-evaluate the research.

(BPS 2004)

Why research that has not been approved is not necessarily unethical

The calls for parity between the disciplines suggest that, for some researchers at least, there is an assumption that research that has not undergone review by an ethics committee is not ethical research. Many social science departments require their research students to complete an ethical declaration prior to commencing data collection, but, as noted by Kent et al. (2002), there is no formal requirement to obtain ethics approval for social research projects. However, rather than viewing the lack of ethics approval with suspicion we should be mindful that the regulatory model is simply that – a model: it is not the panacea.

The brief review of the guidelines for BSA above illustrates how issues such as professional integrity, relations with and responsibility towards research participants, and sponsors or funding bodies are addressed in the social sciences. This includes informed and on-going consent, anonymity, the proper conduct of covert research and privacy. Confidence in such guidelines is demonstrated by organisations such as the National Children's Bureau (NCB) whose own published *Guidelines for Research* (NCB 2003) adopted the BSA Approved Statement of Ethical Practice (but included four additions that related specifically to children). The strength of guidelines such as these is that they aim to nurture researchers who can justify how their whole approach, not just their intent, is based on a clear understanding and decision to work within sound moral principles.

Why ethics approval does not necessarily mean ethical research

In contrast, the adoption of the NHS regulatory model may actually have negative implications for the development of skills in ethical decision-making, particularly for student or novice researchers. This approach is in danger of becoming more of an effective choice from a pick and mix of ethical theories by any given researcher in order to justify their proposed intent before the realities of the fieldwork become apparent. The current COREC process emphasises successful negotiation (perhaps manipulation) in a single instance of an external ethics committee rather than personal responsibility. This means that the skill is actually in the production of the proposal rather than the conduct of the study. The assumption is that at the point of scrutiny the researcher's moral decisions have already been made and were acceptable.

Common sense dictates that the ability to comply with the demands of an ethics committee does not address the possibility that a researcher may have to respond to unforeseen events and ethical issues that cannot be predicted and included in REC review. The REC system has no function in ensuring that recommendations are pursued following approval, and it has been argued that this would not be appropriate or feasible in any case (Pickworth 2000). If this is the case, then we will always rely on the researchers themselves to carry out their proposed study in an ethical way, which means that self-regulation is a necessity that cannot be circumvented or overridden.

If discussion, deliberation and education are the key to ethical research then opportunities to engage in such activity should be available to researchers not only at the initial stages of their research, but throughout. In the regulatory model, the main business of ethics takes place within the committee before fieldwork begins, which obviously limits the opportunity for debating and discussing tricky ethical issues. Furthermore, it could be argued that personal integrity in research relies to some extent on socialisation into a research community that is being compromised through the limitations on the research opportunities for students. This presents us with a very real danger that future opportunities for development of these skills may dwindle due to the emphasis on 'getting through ethics approval'.

The ethics committee, however well intentioned, cannot always engage sufficiently with the intricacies of a researcher's methodological approach. Halse and Honey (2005) demonstrate this most effectively with their explanation of how compliance with an ethics committee's demands did not necessarily make for ethical research as defined by themselves as feminist researchers. Issues they faced about the contrasting descriptions of anorexia used by the medical staff and their intended participants created moral problems for them that were not entirely understood by the ethics committee scrutinising their proposal. Throughout their deliberations they maintain that compliance is nurtured when a stalemate is reached between the committee and the researcher, and that through this the possibility arises that 'cultures of counterfeit practice' (p. 2142) are cultivated.

Personal responsibility and peer review as a means to ensure ethical research

Reliance on the acceptance of personal responsibility alone would present only a limited means to ensure ethical research. The researcher would remain isolated and bereft of external input into their deliberations, and third-party surveillance of deliberate or inadvertent unethical behaviour would be lost (even the limited prospective review provided by the REC approach). Alderson warns of this potential isolationism, though her solution is for greater social researcher involvement in RECs. In response to the problems that abound in the REC system she suggests that:

> *Research communities may decide that these problems are irresolvable, and that informal review by an individual or a small group, or no review at all, is preferable. However, this means that social research is conducted amid unresolved problems about ethics, with little or no formal protection for research subjects, or for the reputation of social research and of research institutions. Individuals or small group review can repeat the faults of the least efficient RECs, with the added problems that they can be more arbitrary and secretive.*
> (Alderson 1995, p. 39)

If the scenario that Alderson portrays were widespread then it would, indeed, give cause for grave concern. Fortunately, personal responsibility is only one part of the process.

Peer review

Peer review indicates critical appraisal of intended research by research colleagues who are equally committed to engaging only in ethically acceptable research practice. (In the case of research students peer review should be undertaken with senior colleagues and supervisors.) It involves deep, prolonged discussion to ensure that issues are fully analysed and a variety of solutions considered (as compared to a severely time-limited review by committee). Rather than an adversarial scenario in which the researcher tries to persuade others of their viewpoint, peer review engages the researcher in self-critique and review of their beliefs and judgements in a supportive environment. Solutions are arrived at in a timely, context-specific manner with due regard for the interests of the specific participant. This may be done more generally in health research, but it is not often reported and is not as transparent as in this system where discussion with colleagues would be expected in reasonable proximity to the event.

Most formal internal review processes, such as university research ethics and governance committee review, fail to offer the *peer* part of peer review and are likely to be more concerned with protecting the finances and good name of the university. Alternative formal approaches are to be found, however. In Australia, for example, 'institutional ethics officers', who are specialists in research ethics policy, act as consultants for researchers who need to discuss ethical difficulties or research dilemmas before the proposal is put before a review committee (Halse & Honey 2005). This also protects the confidentiality of members of ethics committees and reduces the possibilities of manipulation.

CONCLUSION

Adopting the REC system as the sole and essential guarantor of ethical conduct in research is, therefore, flawed for three main reasons. First, it is no guarantee of ethical research. Moreover, it denies the possibility of an alternative approach in cases not susceptible to scrutiny by a NHS REC. This is to the detriment of the work of individuals pursuing such an approach and damages the potential for implementation and dissemination. Finally, it risks missing the benefit of the development in researchers of a mindset and capability to think beyond the rules and prescribed requirements of unresponsive codes, to identify solutions to non-standard ethical problems and to react appropriately when an immediate response is needed in the field. The latter ability is achieved only through prior review of numerous theoretical possibilities, leading to the formulation and internalisation of key principles to guide actions in anomalous situations.

'Key principles' in this sense does not refer to what has sometimes been disparagingly termed 'The Georgetown Mantra' of respect for autonomy, beneficence, non-maleficence and justice. These often-quoted but poorly-understood concepts are often too simplistic for tackling the complexity of ethical issues in practice and in research. The principles conflict far too easily, for example, notably when attempting to act in someone's best interests when they make unwise, capricious decisions while also trying to respect their autonomy. Another approach that fails to provide sufficient responsiveness to the complex reality of health and social care is the adoption of inflexible codes of ethical conduct (rather than the more flexible guidance offered by the BPS and the BSA). These become more and more convoluted as qualifying additions are made to cater for exceptions to rules and atypical cases that they become impossibly unwieldy, making conflicting demands on the researcher and ultimately providing no guidance for the researcher's own critical judgement on the specific case or circumstances at issue.

In this chapter we have argued that approval is not a guarantee of ethical research, the lack of approval from a REC does not automatically equate to unethical research, and compliance with the REC system is no indicator of ethical decision-making ability or practice. The over-simplicity of the quest for 'approval' disguises a lack of recognition of the more important activity of on-going ethical decision-making. The REC system may be leading us into an era of unthinking research in the ethical domain in which the REC 'nanny' does the thinking for researchers, and a bland menu of options is offered that fails to reflect the complex reality of research in health and social care. When review by a NHS REC is available and required, then it should be pursued, but this does not absolve the researcher of responsibility for identifying and addressing ethical issues before and after formal ethics approval. Whether REC approval is required or not, re-emphasis of personal responsibility and the adoption of peer review does much more to support and strengthen this endeavour.

REFERENCES

Alderson P (1995) Listening to children: children, ethics and social research, Barnardos, Ilford.

British Psychological Society (2004) Ethical principles for conducting research with human participants. BPS, London.

British Sociological Association (2002) Statement of ethical practice for the British Sociological Association. BSA, London.

Community Practitioners' and Health Visitors' Association, Royal College of Midwives and Royal College of Nursing (2005) A position paper on the implementation of research governance procedures. CPHVA, London.

Coomber R (2002) Signing your life away? Why research ethics committees (REC) shouldn't always require written confirmation that participants in research have been informed of the aims of a study and their rights - the case of criminal populations (Commentary). Sociological Research Online 7(1). http://www.socresonline.org.uk/7/1/coomber.html

Department of Health (1991) Local Research Ethics Committees (HSG(91)5). DH, London.

Department of Health (2001) Research governance framework for health and social care. DH, London.

Department of Health (2005) Report of an ad hoc advisory group on the operation of NHS research ethics committees (Warner Report). DH, London.

Dolan B (1999) The impact of local research ethics committees on the development of nursing knowledge. Journal of Advanced Nursing 30(5), 1009–1010.

Halse C, Honey A (2005) Unravelling Ethics: Illuminating the Moral Dilemmas of Research Ethics. SIGNS: Journal of Women in Culture and Society 30(4), 2141–2162.

Jamrozik K (2000) The case for a new system for oversight of research on human subjects. Journal of Medical Ethics 26(5), 334–339.

Johnson M (1999) Scholarship, namedropping and the '5 minute test'. Nurse Education Today 19(8), 599–600.

Kaur B, Taylor J (1996) Separate criteria should be drawn up for questionnaire based epidemiological studies. British Medical Journal 312(7022), 54b–54.

Kent J, Williamson E, Goodenough T, Ashcroft R (2002) Social science gets the ethics treatment: research governance and ethical review. Sociological Research Online 7(4) http://www.socresonline.org.uk/7/4/williamson.html

Lewis J, Tomkins S, Sampson J (2001) Ethical approval for research involving geographically dispersed subjects: unsuitability of the UK MREC/LREC system and relevance to uncommon genetic disorders. Journal of Medical Ethics 27(5), 347–351.

Lux A, Edwards S, Osborne J (2000) Responses of local research ethics committees to a study with approval from a multicentre research ethics committee. British Medical Journal 320(7243), 1182–1183.

Middle C, Johnson A, Petty T, Sims L, Macfarlane A (1995) Ethics approval for a national postal survey: recent experience. British Medical Journal 311, 659–660.

Nicholson R (ed.) (1986) Medical research with children: ethics, law and practice. Cambridge University Press.

National Children's Bureau (2003) Guidelines for research. http://www.ncb.org.uk/ourwork/research_guidelines.pdf (Accessed 11.01.06)

Oddens B, De Wied D (1995) Committees should devise special forms for the social sciences. British Medical Journal 311(7019), 1572.

Osborn D, Fulford K (2003) Psychiatric research: what ethical concerns do LRECs encounter? A postal survey. Journal of Medical Ethics 29(1), 55–56.

Pappworth M (1967) Human guinea pigs: experimentation on man. Routledge, London.

Pickworth E (2000) Should local research ethics committees monitor research they have approved? Journal of Medical Ethics 26(5), 330–333.

Stone P, Blogg C (1997) Local research ethics committees. British Medical Journal 315, 60–61.

Tod A, Nicolson P, Allmark P (2002) Ethical review of health service research in the UK: implications for nursing. Journal of Advanced Nursing 40(4), 379–386.

10

Techno-research and cyber ethics: research using the Internet[1]

Carol Haigh and Neil Jones

INTRODUCTION

The development of Internet technology over the past decade has seen a corresponding growth in the development and use of Internet-based research methodologies (Elgesem 2003). Although health research has been slow to recognise the advantages of techno-research, there is some evidence that the Internet is now being seen as a useful research resource. The purpose of this chapter is briefly to outline the potential that the World Wide Web has for researchers both as a source of research materials and as a method of collecting data. In the chapter we will also explore some of the common issues of concern surrounding techno-research and will introduce a cyber-ethics framework that will allow techno-researchers to identify the potential threats and hazards inherent in their study. Although the nomenclature of the Internet and Internet research is dynamic and changing, for the sake of consistency throughout this chapter, we will use the phrase techno-research to describe research carried out using electronic media such as the World Wide Web, e-mail, listserv, etc. A techno-researcher is one who plans such research. Cyberspace is taken to mean the virtual as opposed to the 'real' world.

TECHNO-RESEARCH

Internet-based research is reasonably well established in other disciplines such as media studies, sociology and cultural studies.

---

[1] Some of the content of this chapter appeared in Haigh, C Jones NA (2005) An overview of the ethics of cyber-space research and the implications for nurse educators. Nurse Education Today 25(1), 3–8 and is reproduced with kind permission of the Editor

Health-care professions, and nursing in particular, have been slow to exploit the World Wide Web as a data collection tool. The Internet offers clear advantages as a research tool for:

● recruiting and accessing hard-to-research groups
● allowing for geographical spread and richness in data collection,
● providing safe virtual environments for researchers to carry out interviews or focus groups
● allowing for a broader range of sample
(Coomber 1997, Brownlow & O'Dell 2002).

These advantages can be used to enhance research activities and to allow exploration of an under-utilised medium of enquiry. Furthermore, it is a matter of concern when journals continually publish articles purporting to be research that have used the convenience sample of the author's own student, client or patient group. Internet research allows for much wider data collection across disparate groups which share a common experience and in this way contributes to rigorous and *meaningful* research that is generalisable to more than one institution, or even more than one country.

Using the Internet as source material

The first stage of any research study is to explore the current literature within that topic (Bowling 2002). A truly comprehensive literature review will take into account both published and unpublished work and in the past this has been a time consuming element of the research process with long hours being spent in the library. Using the Internet means that library catalogues (from virtually any library in the world) can be searched for source material in a fraction of the time. Additionally, a number of full text resources will be available via journal, newspaper and periodicals databases and a number of classical methodological and philosophical texts can be accessed free of charge at the Project Gutenberg web site or at the On-line Books Page.[2] On line literature searchers can also access government websites and statistical databases at national and international level (Hewson et al. 2003).

---

[2] Since Internet Domains and web site addresses change rapidly it is not seen as useful to provide a URL for these sites. However, putting these titles as search terms in a meta search engine such as google.com will find the page quickly

One of the difficulties that beset any literature searcher is that of tracing 'grey literature'. In the UK, unpublished PhD theses relevant to nursing can be accessed by a personal visit to the Steinberg Collection of the Royal College of Nursing. Works in other health disciplines can be obtained via an inter-library loan from the British Library. Other grey literature, such as internal research reports, may never be available to the literature searcher. However, the Internet allows for these primary sources to be accessed with relative ease if they are available by this route.

Using the Internet to collect data

Hewson et al. (2003) have conservatively estimated that there are over 195 countries with international Internet connectivity and that the Internet user population exceeds the 500 million mark. This suggests that the Internet can be a significant source of data. A number of established exploratory methods lend themselves to Internet research and, although they are not new, they allow for new perspectives on established information gathering techniques to be used (Coomber 1997). Suitable methods for use in Internet research include:

- web-page content analysis
- on-line focus groups
- on-line interviews
- analysis of 'e' conversation.

Observational techniques can be used in electronic communities. Brownlow and O'Dell (2002) note the advantages afforded to the non-participant observer in chat rooms by 'lurking': entering the chat room but not participating. Overt participation in synchronous chat rooms (cyberspace areas where interactions take place in real time) can be carried out without the confounding variables associated with race, gender or age, which may be seen as an advantage. Additionally, asynchronous listservs or newsgroups (sites where messages are posted but interaction does not take place in real time) can allow in-depth analysis of content.

CYBER-ETHICS

Many of the concerns that exercise cyber-ethicists are those of 'real-world' research. These include concepts such as ensuring confidentiality and privacy of respondents, gathering informed consent from participants and the prevention of harm (Jankowski & van Slem 2001). That these are issues of joint concern to both techno and real-world researchers is conceded; however, certain issues require greater consideration in cyber-space than is generally expected from human subject research not involving the Internet (Association of Internet Researchers 2002). The Association of Internet Researchers (AoIR) felt that there was greater difficulty surrounding privacy and confidentiality, informed consent and ascertaining the identity of subjects. It was further acknowledged that, as Internet research was global in scope, extra consideration should be given to the best eclectic ethical approach. The guidelines contrast the primarily utilitarian ethical stance of research in the USA with the chiefly deontological approach that is fundamental in European research (AoIR 2002). Overall, ethical pluralism is suggested as a compromise to the differing global ethical approaches. The AoIR report stopped short of a specific Internet ethics framework, preferring to reinforce the underpinning tenets of all research, real or virtual; respect for persons and protection from harm. In the light of this it makes sense to argue that the Internet is now part of the 'real world'.

It is these tenets that have informed much of the debate surrounding Internet research ethics (Jankowski & van Selm 2001, Bruckman 2002a), and the human subject research model has become the main ethical model contributing to the ethics of on-line research. Bassett and O'Riorden (2002) attempted to depose this model by taking the stance that focussing upon the human players was to miss the significant 'textuality' of the Internet. They argued that, since the Internet is a cultural production with a framework similar to that of print media, broadcast television and radio, it must be viewed in the same way. The crux of Bassett and O'Riorden's argument is that the arguments of privacy and safety that are central to the human subject model of Internet ethics can eclipse other equally important textual concepts such as representation and publication of ideas. An illustrative example of this would be the decision to ignore the archive newsgroup postings of individuals who had left the discussion list and so could not give their consent. By omitting their ideas and opinions significant data may be lost to a study.

On the other hand, Bruckman (2002a) argues from a strict 'informed consent' standpoint, although she does allow that, for some researchers, a less rigorous and more fluid approach may be appropriate. Like the AoIR (2002), Bruckman puts the ethical decision-making inherent in Internet research firmly back upon the shoulders of the researcher themselves, offering no more than a framework for discussion. Nonetheless, the framework offered by Bruckman does provide triggers for the ethical evaluation of proposed Internet research projects. The primary concerns and key dilemmas for techno-researchers are as follows.

Analysis of on-line information

No information published on the World Wide Web is copyright free. We support the stance of Bruckman (2002a) who suggests that information may only be used and subjected to analytical techniques if it is (i) publicly archived, (ii) the archives are not password protected or do not require you to register with the site to gain access, (iii) the site policy does not prohibit it and (iv) the topic is not highly sensitive (Haigh & Jones 2005).

Consent

Consent needs to be considered. It may be obtained electronically if the respondent is over 18 years old, but this is only appropriate if the risk to participants is low and if the on-line consent form takes potential participants through the documentation a step at a time. Additionally, the consent process must not be perceived as disruptive to discourse in the virtual world that the researcher chooses to use (Haigh & Jones 2005).

If consent is being sought from minors, parental consent must be obtained in paper format (via surface mail or fax) or verbally if the research is low risk. If the on-line researcher wishes to interview minors on-line then parental consent must be obtained in a face-to-face interview (Bruckman 2002a).

Privacy and confidentiality

In contrast to the USA, European citizens enjoy stringent levels of personal data security thanks to the European Union Data Protection Directive (1995). This means that participants should be protected from having their data transferred to countries with less rigorous levels of protection of privacy (AoIR 2002).

The on-line researcher needs to consider, in some detail, how they are obtaining their data and how the venue in which the data is collected is viewed. The main locations of this concern are those of chat rooms or newsgroups. It can be argued that a chat room can be viewed as if it were a public place like a staff room or a restaurant.

However, Waskul (1996) suggests that definitions of 'public' and 'private' do not translate so neatly to cyberspace. He argues that cyberspace defies locality and that on-line interaction cannot be defined as either public or private, but both public and private. He goes on to put forward the view that 'public' and 'private' are mere metaphors when applied to cyberspace. This argument arises from the fact that individuals may engage in public on-line interactions, whilst in the privacy of their own homes. Waskul likens the situation to individuals having a private discussion in a public place (for example a park bench), while a researcher secretly records their conversation. He supports his argument further by citing King's (1995) assertion that the nature of on-line interactions gives rise to a false perception of greater privacy. Therefore, on-line environments, which are described as 'public', may not necessarily match the social definition of that environment.

Even if we argue that it is acceptable to obtain data from such public/private domains provided consent is obtained and the individual is not identifiable, this is not necessarily a practical option in Internet research when recording an ephemeral interaction, such as chat room conversation. The posting of messages asking for participant consent may be disruptive to the very activity that the researcher is interested in.

The need to disguise the identity of subjects needs to be clarified prior to commencing the research. It can be argued that most chat room users have already created pseudonyms for themselves, which makes identity concealment by the researcher less necessary. However, in the virtual world pseudonyms function in a manner analogous to real names and should be treated as such. Bruckman (2002a) states that this is because the pseudonym is often traceable to a real name and also because people care about the reputation of their pseudonym as much as they do about their real name. To facilitate this Bruckman outlines four levels of, what she terms, 'disguise' that can be applied to Internet study participants:

1. **No disguise:** If we accept Bassett and O'Riorden's (2002) stance that the textual richness of the Internet must be recognized as a legitimate data source, then the right of individuals to be credited with the material they have created is evident. This ensures that copyright claims are respected, but does place an onus upon the researcher to verify authorship, which is not always as overt in web-based materials as in the traditional paper-based products.
2. **Light disguise:** Allows for the group used to be named, although pseudonyms are changed. Nonetheless, group members may be able to identify each other when the data is

presented. Verbatim quotes are used, even if they could be used to identify an individual.

3. **Moderate disguise:** is a compromise between light disguise and complete disguise and must be carefully and fully considered at the ethical permission stage of the study.

4. **Complete disguise:** All is concealed; group name and pseudonyms so that subjects are not recognizable either to themselves or to a third party. No verbatim quotations are used if these would facilitate group identity via a search engine. Bruckman (2002a) argues that some deliberately false details may be introduced, changing the name of the disease being studied for example, but it must be stressed that this approach is not without ethical problems of its own. In such a case it should be clear to all what factors have been re-labelled and why.

It must be emphasised that, regardless of the level of disguise chosen, any details that would be harmful to the participants should be omitted from publication. The only possible exception to this is the level of complete disguise, which if carried out rigorously, will allow details that are potentially harmful to subjects to be published since their identity is completely obscured. Coupled with and impacted upon by issues of privacy and cyber-personality is the need to debrief research participants whilst at the same time protecting their privacy. Traditional approaches to data collection usually involve a face-to-face verbal explanation of the study and an invitation to the participant to ask questions or make further comment. Additionally, the researcher can reassure themselves that the participant has not suffered any harm or distress from the research procedure. This type of interaction is compromised by techno-research. Hewson et al. (2003) suggest the sending of a 'de-briefing text' that provides some explanation of the purpose of the study and the contact details of the researcher should further information be required. This message can be sent either via a web browser or in an e-mail immediately after the participant has submitted their responses.

Thus far, the ethical components of techno-research that we have considered have been those that have counterparts in traditional (non-Internet-based) research. However, there are exceptional aspects of cyberspace that can impact upon the ethical foundations of research in ways that are unique to the medium. These aspects include issues of 'disinhibition' and 'virtual persona'.

Disinhibition

A number of writers have commented on the disinhibiting effects of cyberspace (Chandler & Roberts-Young 1998, Bruckman 2002b, Suler 2004). Generally, people are more prepared to share secrets, personal information and express themselves more openly in on-line environments. It has been noted that disinhibition is often associated with the degree of anonymity afforded by the various virtual environments and the potential for concealment of real-world identity associated with the increasing immersion in the virtual world (Suler 2004).

Chandler (1997) points out that authors of personal home pages avoid using assumed identities that are unrecognisable to those who know them. So anonymity tends not to be an issue at this level. However, even at the superficial level of the home page, where real-world identity is most accessible, the phenomenon of disinhibition is also observed. For example, Chandler (1998) recounts how one gay man 'came out' in cyberspace through the medium of his personal web page before being out in the real world.

Disinhibition, in part, is a function of invisibility. Even though an individual's identity may be known to other inhabitants of cyber-space, the fact that they cannot see or be seen in the virtual setting enhances the effect. This disinhibition may be further supported by the asynchronous nature of e-mail and message boards and lack of non-verbal cues from others (Chandler 1998, Suler 2004). On the face of it this is of advantage to the researcher in terms of subject compliance and increased self-disclosure in providing information. However, Bruckman (2002b) stresses that the researcher has clear ethical responsibility to protect the individual by preserving anonymity even when the participant does not share this concern. This paternalistic approach to techno-research participants is seen in the work of Chandler and Roberts-Young (1998) who, in their study of personal home pages of adolescents, protected minors from excessive self-revelation by omitting sensitive but voluntarily disclosed details from subsequent publications.

Suler (2004) describes a number of manifestations of on-line disinhibition. In addition to the benign sharing of information and inner secrets, disinhibition may take the form of rudeness, anger and harsh criticism. This behaviour may contrast sharply with the person's real-world personality. It can vary from the relatively harmless use of provocative or angry e-mails (flaming) to the propensity of some individuals to explore what Suler calls 'the dark underworld of the Internet', which includes violent or pornographic web sites. This may be due in part to users being able to separate their actions from their real-world identity. The individual does not have to take responsibility for their behaviour and can, therefore, dissociate themselves from their actions.

The creation of an imaginary cyberspace persona also contributes to disinhibited behaviour. In isolation individuals may feel that the on-line persona and members of their virtual community exist in a make believe dimension. Suler states that this can be seen as a dream world, which separates the individual from real-world norms. Although some people suggest that the disinhibiting effect allows the emergence of the true self, Suler rejects this claim asserting that the notion of a true self is too ambiguous to serve as a useful concept. The philosophical debate that is attendant upon this notion is one that researchers may care to participate in. The ambiguity of the true self could be argued to be a confounding variable of all, not just techno, research.

Nonetheless, the disinhibition effect has very real implications for research and cyberspace research ethics. If it arises as a result of fantasy, dreaming or an altered state of consciousness, we must question its relevance to real-world, every-day consciousness and how this may impact upon any research study. The potential degree of disinhibition and its implications for both the accuracy of the data and appropriateness of informed consent must be considered. The ethical considerations relate to whether on-line disinhibition is likely to put the participant, or others, at risk in the real world.

Cyberspace persona, avatars and pseudonyms

Concealment of real-world identity in virtual settings is a common practice and as one moves progressively through the layers of cyberspace real-world identities become more obscured. Physical attributes, age, sex and gender are unclear and lack of certainty regarding individual 'real-world' characteristics presents quite obvious problems to the researcher. Concealment may include strategies such as gender switching (Chandler 1998, Suler 1999a), the use of pseudonyms (Bruckman 2002a) or the use of 'avatars'.

The term avatar has its origin in the Hindu tradition and relates to the earthly manifestation of a god. The concept has been adopted in cyberspace to provide a visual representation of the person. These pictorial images are attached to individual text contributions. Avatars vary in design from simple graphic designs to intricate fantasy images. They may be human images, pictures of animals or take more abstract forms. Avatars may be animated or static images. They are also used to support gender switching in some virtual settings when an individual adopts the opposite gender as their on-line persona. So, a male may use a female name and a female avatar. The phenomenon of gender switching is apparently quite common in some Internet communities (not all of them sexually focussed). Though some women try gender switching, it is more common among men (Suller 1999a). The levels of anonymity offered by an avatar are so strong and the gender switch so convincing that other group members are often unaware of the switcher's real-world gender.

An important point about avatars is that, like pseudonyms, they are regarded as part of the individual's cyber identity. Suler (1999b) relates how members of one on-line group would ostracise anyone who dared to use someone else's avatar. The on-line persona can be very convincing and perceived as authentic, even by other members of the virtual community. This highlights potential difficulties that the researcher may face when trying to ascertain a participant's real-world attributes in a virtual setting.

Techno-researchers should question whether personality disguise, such as that afforded by avatars, pose a threat to the integrity of the research per se and whether there are measures that can be planned into the research to protect the integrity of the data. Suler's (1999a) questionnaire to discriminate between women and gender-switching men was designed by women and focusses exclusively upon female biology and feminine products, and is an example of such measures.

HOW CAN POTENTIAL ETHICAL PROBLEMS OF TECHNO-RESEARCH BE ADDRESSED?

As with other forms of research, the aim of techno-research is to protect the wellbeing of the subject by minimising risks. The integrity of the research depends upon this and validity of the research depends upon the reliability and veracity of the data. To a greater or lesser extent, some areas of cyberspace pose potential risks to both the wellbeing of participants and the integrity of the research.

It is clear that the most effective way to address potential ethical problems in any techno-research project is to identify them before starting. The difficulty with this approach is that ethical frameworks other than those that are established in 'real-world research' are non-directive, putting the burden firmly on the shoulders of the researcher. Given the relatively meagre experience that most health care researchers have with this particular method of inquiry, this burden may be onerous.

In real-world settings individuals react to and interact with their environment. The same holds true for the virtual settings of the Internet. The ethical impact grid (Fig. 10.1) identifies the different levels of ethical concern that pose potential threats to either the participants or to the overall integrity of the research and can be utilised to assess the ethical impact of techno-research methods.

The ethical dimensions of environment, participant identity, privacy, data reliability, research methods and ethical dilemmas are based upon the elements of concern identified within the AoIR guidelines for Internet research ethics (2002). These headings represent key factors in cyberspace research, how they impact on each other and the resulting level of ethical concern. The Internet and cyberspace are merely convenient terms for a variety of electronically mediated communication methods. The ethical impact grid presents them as different environments in cyberspace. These include:

- Public: This includes publicly accessible domains such as personal web pages. Typically these areas of cyber-space have open access and no entry restrictions.
- Semi-public: These areas include communication methods such as e-mail or free to register websites that require a

Figure 10.1 Ethical impact grid

Levels	Environment	Participant ID	Privacy	Data reliability	Research methods	Ethical dilemmas
1	Public (e.g. web space)	Accessible real world ID	None	Strong	Neutral	Superficial
2	Semi-public (e.g. e-mail)	Controlled real world ID	Light	Strong	Overt participation	Minimal
3	Semi-private (e.g. listserv)	Accessible virtual world ID	Light moderate	Moderate	Overt non-participation	Moderate
4	Private (e.g. Chatroom)	Controlled virtual world ID	Moderate	Weak	Covert participation	Significant
5	Virtual (role-playing)	Complete virtual world immersion	Heavy	Unreliable	Covert non-participation	Highly significant

superficial amount of knowledge, such as the e-mail address of individuals or a user name and password, but which have little or no entry restrictions upon them.

- Semi-private: Refers to cyber environments, such as listserv, a programme that automatically sends e-mail to subscribers of a mailing list. Mailings are aimed at specialist interest groups or specific professions, they require registration (sometimes with payment), and are not easily accessible to non-members.
- Private: This cyber-environment is one in which membership is exclusive, but generally focussed upon many topics. Virtual alliances can be forged and newcomers are recognised as such. Users of this level can switch persona easily and avatar use is common, e.g. chat rooms.
- Virtual: This is the deepest level of cyber-space immersion where 'real-world' persona holds no sway and fantasy is commonplace, e.g. role playing.

From the perspective of the techno-researcher the engagement of the Internet user/potential research participant with cyberspace's many domains can represent different levels of immersion. Moving down through the successive levels from one to five we find greater immersion in cyberspace culture and less certainty with regard to real-world, face-to-face identity. The degree of risk to research participants and, therefore, the ethical considerations, vary between each area.

As with any tool the ethical impact grid has limitations and can act only as a guide to ethical considerations. It is not intended to be a substitute for the researcher's power of reasoning and an understanding of ethical principles is essential. It will be necessary for the researcher to adapt and apply as individual circumstances dictate.

Level 1

The focus of level 1 is the public environment of the web page. The subjects, content and style of web pages are many and varied. They include the professional, the corporate and the personal. The authors tend to be identifiable and anonymity is generally not an issue (Chandler 1997). Suitable research methods at this level include web page content analysis.

Ethical considerations are minimal but web pages should be cited and referenced as other sources of literature, as previously mentioned. The difficulty here is that web page content is often highly derivative and it is not always easy to trace the original source. Eysenbach (2000) suggests that plagiarism of website content is a problem that is on the increase. Bruckman (2000a) considers it to be the researcher's responsibility to ensure the acknowledgement of the original author.

Level 2

In the semi-public environment of e-mail, level 2 may merge with level 3 to some extent. This depends on the participants and how they are recruited. E-mail is a commonly used method of communication. It lends itself readily to surveys of respondents likely to have e-mail services and when targeted carefully the researcher can be quite certain of the credentials and identity of the recipients. At least this is the case in targeting organised groups such as hospital or university staff, members of professional bodies or employees who have access to a company e-mail address. In this situation there is a degree of organisational control concerning network use and the assigning of e-mail addresses.

However, if a researcher were to attempt to target a wider population, by canvassing visitors to a website, for example, there would not be the same degree of certainty of the identity. It is also very likely that many of the e-mail addresses would contain pseudonyms and this highlights the further threat to the integrity of the research since the credentials of the respondents would likewise not be obvious. The self-selecting respondents come with a degree of anonymity. In this respect there is overlap with level 3 of the grid.

Research methods suitable for e-mail are surveys or interviews. These can be carried out by means of electronic questionnaires or electronic one-to-one interview by e-mail. Whichever method is used, the techno-researcher is overtly participative and may direct the researcher/respondent interaction. The problem of self selection leaves the survey/interview subject to selection bias, i.e. a non-representative sample. The main ethical concerns of this level relate to the difficulties of obtaining informed consent and anonymity.

Level 3

Level 3 deals with the listserv. This environment is semi private with real-world identity possibly (though not necessarily) slightly obscured by the use of a pseudonym in the e-mail address. The decreased certainty over the real-world identity of the participants means there is less confidence in the reliability of the data. A suitable research method for this level is electronic questionnaire.

The primary ethical concerns centre on informed consent issues and the dilemmas that are attendant upon non-participation.

Level 4

The environments designated as 'private' at level 4 include chat rooms. Access is usually password controlled and it is the standard practice to use pseudonyms in these areas.

The ethical considerations are significant at this level. There is in some ways a conflict between protection of participants and the integrity of the research. The real-world identity is obscured. This negatively affects the confidence in data reliability. Eysenbach and Wyatt (2002) point out that the observer effect will possibly change the behaviour of the group in such environments. Therefore, the act of seeking informed consent is likely to influence the results, unless the researcher is willing to accept consent from a cyber persona rather than a 'real-world' identity.

One of the most successful research methods for this setting is covert participation. This method raises ethical concerns as it involves an element of deception. However, a number of authors, notably Johnson (2003, 2004) have argued that the ethical dilemma of deception should be balanced against firstly the risk of harm (which if Bruckman's levels of disguise are applied may be minimal) and, secondly, a comprehensive understanding of the good that may accrue from carrying out the research in secret. Researchers in this situation can approach the group moderator for permission to approach the group to explain the proposed research and sound out reactions. Although the potential for reactive effect (changing behaviour when under observation also known as the Hawthorne effect) must be acknowledged, Clark and Bowling (1990) point out that observed participants in the real world quickly revert to 'normal' behaviour. We can speculate that, in the anonymity of cyberspace, the sense of being under observation may be even more fleeting. The risk of disinhibition can be seen at this level of immersion and may justify a paternalistic approach even if covert participation is undertaken.

Level 5

At level 5 the environment has been described as 'virtual'. These include the games and role-playing areas where we are most likely to find the greatest level of immersion in the virtual world.

Real-world identity is deeply obscured, disinhibition is strong and data unreliable. Research methods available would include covert participation. As discussed above, this has its attendant ethical problems. Unless the techno-researcher is very skilled, however, it is likely that they will quickly be identified by the cyberspace community as 'not one of us'. Not only would this have serious consequences for the entire research project, the risk of harm to participants in their cyber-persona if not their real world one is high. An alternative option would be covert non-participation (lurking); however, this is a most ethically dubious approach and not recommended except in the most extreme circumstances.

POTENTIAL ETHICAL ISSUES IN OBTAINING APPROVAL FOR TECHNO-RESEARCH

In earlier chapters the strategies that a researcher can employ to facilitate ethical approval are outlined. It must be emphasised that techno-research may require extra ethical consideration not least because health-related ethics committees are not overly familiar with cyberspace placed research. So far we have outlined the prime ethical concerns that are attendant upon techno-research and provided an ethical impact grid as a method of organising ethical evaluation of potential projects. In this final section we will attempt to highlight some of the concerns that ethics committees may have.

Consent

Bruckman (2002a) and the AoIR (2002) have provided very clear guidelines upon how informed consent can be obtained from the participants of techno-research. The issues that may exercise ethical approval committees will centre upon validation of identity and the role of the virtual persona.

Vulnerable groups

If study participants are recruited from cyberspace there is a possibility that some will fall within the ubiquitous category of 'vulnerable group'. Although it may be difficult for an ethics committee to understand the notion that members of such groups could be included in the study without the techno-researcher's knowledge, the ethical principle of respect for autonomy would suggest that an individual's informed decision to participate is valid. In other words, we may normally be justified in assuming that, irrespective of qualifying in the real world as 'vulnerable', such vulnerability may be partially overcome by the resources of the Internet and both allow and promote autonomy. On the other hand, the exploitation of young people has provoked particular fears for their safety.

Distressed participants

We have highlighted the difficulty in arranging de-brief interviews in cyber space, and support of research participants who become distressed is likewise difficult. Access to both on-line and traditional support mechanisms should be arranged if the risk of participant distress is calculated to be significant. If the risk of distress is highly likely, techno-research is not the appropriate medium of enquiry.

CONCLUSION

It is clear that the world of cyber space holds opportunities for health researchers that have not this far been fully explored. The contribution that the World Wide Web can make to the access to research participants or the obtaining of cross border/continent opinion, attitude or behaviour is one that cannot be underestimated. Although there are a number of ethical concerns inherent in techno-research that overlap with traditional research, the virtual nature of cyberspace means that greater consideration must be given to such concerns if the research participants, the techno-researcher and the research itself are to be protected. Overlapping concerns include issues such as consent and confidentiality.

Additionally, there are a number of ethical concerns that are unique to cyberspace including the potential for disinhibition and the effects that such behaviour could have not only upon participants or researchers, but also upon the rigour and validity of research data. Sensitivity to the representation of cyber persona and the disguise element of avatar use also impact upon the management and ethical components of techno-research.

This ethical impact grid that we present in this chapter is designed to help novice researchers consider the ethical dimensions that underpin the different layers of cyber space, the methodological approaches to information gathering and the amount of immersion that can be expected from the cyber-residents. It is not intended to replace basic ethical considerations, but to supplement them within this specific domain and to provide a foundation for deliberation before commencing upon Internet-based research of any sort.

Finally, it must also be remembered that good Internet research is anchored within the overall social context and should, ideally therefore, have an off-line component to complement the on-line data collection.

REFERENCES

Association of Internet Researchers (2002) Ethical decision making and internet research. Recommendations from the AoIR ethics working committee.
www.aoir.org/report/ethics/pdf (accessed 06/08/03)

Bowling A (2002) Research methods in health. Investigating health and health services. Open University Press. Buckingham

Brownlow C, O'Dell L (2002) Ethical Issues for qualitative research in on-line communities. Disability and Society 17, 685–694.

Bruckman A (2002a) Ethical guidelines for research online.
http://www.cc.atech.edu/~asb/ethics/ (accessed 08/07/03)

Bruckman A (2002b) Studying the amateur artist: a perspective on disguised data collected in human subjects research on the internet.
http://www.nyu.edu?projects/nissenbaum/ethics_bru_full.html (accessed 06/03/05)

Chandler D (1997) Writing Oneself in Cyberspace.
http://www. aber.ac.uk/media/Documents/short/homepigd.html (accessed 13/04/05)

Chandler D (1998) Personal home pages and the construction of identities on the web.
http://www.aber.ac.uk?media/Documents/short/webident.html (accessed 13/04/05)

Chandler D, Roberts-Young D (1998) The construction of identity in the personal homepages of adolescents.
http://www.aber.ac.uk/media/Documents/short/strasbourg (accessed 13/04/05)

Clark P, Bowling A (1990) Quality of everyday life in long stay institutions for the elderly. An observational study of long stay hospital and nursing home care. Social Science and Medicine 30, 1201–1210

Coomber R (1997) Using the internet for survey research: Sociological Research Online.
http://www.socresonline.org.uk/socresonline/2/2/2.html (accessed 01/08/03)

Elgesem D (2003) What is so special about the ethical issues in on line research: Internet Research Ethics?
http://www.nyu.edu/projects/nissenbaum/ethics_elg_full.html (accessed 08/07/03)

European Union (1995) Directive 95/46/EC of the European Parliament and of the Council of 24 October 1995 on the protection of individuals with regard to the processing of personal data and on the free movement of such data.

http://www.cdt.org/privacy/eudirective/EU_Directive.html
(Accessed 24/05/05)

Eysenbach G (2002) Report of a case of cyberplagiarism - and
reflections on detecting and preventing academic misconduct using
the internet. Journal of Medical Internet Research 2(1):e4 (online)
http://www.jmir.org/2000/1/e4/ (accessed 19/06/05)

Eysenbach G, Wyatt J (2002) Using the internet for surveys and health
research. Journal of Medical Internet Research 4(2):e13 (online)
http://www.jmir.org/2002/2/e13/ (accessed 13/04/05)

Haigh C, Jones NA (2005) An overview of the ethics of cyber-space
research and the implications for nurse educators. Nurse Education
Today 25(1), 3–8.

Hewson C, Yule P, Laurent D, Vogel C (2003) Internet Research
Methods. A practical guide for the social and behavioural sciences.
Sage Publications. London

Jankowski N, van Selm M (2001) Research ethics in a virtual world:
some guidelines and illustrations.
http://www.brunel.ac.uk/depts/crict/vmpapers/nick.htm
(accessed 17/06/03)

Johnson M (2003) Research ethics and education; a consequentialist
view. Nurse Education Today 23, 165–167.

Johnson M (2004) Real-world ethics and nursing research. Journal of
Research in Nursing 9, 251–261.

Suler J (1999a) Do boys (and girls) just wanna have fun? Gender-
switching in cyberspace.
http://www.rider.edu/~suler/psycyber/genderswap.html (accessed
03/03/05)

Suler J (1999b) The psychology of avatars and graphical space in
multimedia chat communities.
http://www.rider.edu/~suler/psycyber/psyav.html#Personal
(accessed 03/03/03)

Suler J (2004) The online disinhibition effect.
http://www.rider.edu/~suler/psycber/disinhibit.html (accessed
03/03/05)

Waskul D (1996) Ethics of online research: considerations for the study
of computer mediated forms of interaction.
http://venus.soci.niu.edu/~jthomas/ethics/tis/go.dennis (accessed
30/11/03)

11

Ethical issues of intervention in research

Martin Johnson

INTRODUCTION

In this chapter[1] I will argue that nurses and other health- and social-care researchers have paid little or no attention to the concept of intervention, despite the fact that it is a key concept in both experimental and qualitative studies. Intervention in any or all of its forms is somehow neglected. I am concerned here to identify the nature of intervention, the conditions under which it is necessary, and why it is particularly problematic from an ethical standpoint.

For health and social care professionals an intervention is a planned act or acts of treatment or care that are based upon an assessment of client need. Nurses, for example, have described a key stage of their 'nursing process', by which care is planned and executed, as the intervention phase. This would normally be identified in writing in advance (Kratz et al. 1979). In another sense, intervention is an action delivered quickly, some would say intuitively, in response to an unexpected need for care (Street 1992). My aim here is to investigate both types of intervention within the context of research of various kinds.

INTERVENTION: THE EXPERIMENTALIST VIEW

Researchers who carry a predominantly positivist view of the world feel bound to make two assumptions about the nature of interventions as they might occur in health and social care research:

- The only interventions that happen should be 'medical' and should have been carefully planned.

---

[1] This chapter is developed from a paper first published as Johnson M (1997) Observations on the neglected concept of intervention in nursing research. Journal of Advanced Nursing 25, 23–29.

- Ideally, there should be no interventions in non-medical research.

In relation to the first it is clear that university, local and multi-centre research ethics committees (RECs) can operate effectively only upon the premise that all aspects of the research have been planned in advance and are identified in the research proposal that they have before them. Large-scale medical clinical trials often reach this level of apparent sophistication where a series of 'if.......then' statements can be included in the protocol. That is to say if, following an intervention such as a drug treatment the research participant gets an allergy, their membership of the study sample can be terminated and perhaps medical treatment can be prescribed. In some cases therapeutic counselling might even be built in and resourced within the trial. Thus, on this model, interventions of all types are planned.

Medical trials are commonly resourced by multinational drug companies who can stand large liability claims because they are heavily insured. For this reason RECs can take this into account when allowing potentially harmful agents, such as anti-cancer drugs to be used as interventions with their clients. Whether this is ethics or economics is an interesting question.

The second assumption is becoming more prevalent in the modern health service context where 'hygienic' forms of research prevail. By these I mean questionnaires and semi-structured interviews that are commonly undertaken with samples of convenience such as student nurses (Bradby 1990). It seems that non-medical students of research are often dissuaded from any kind of contact with patients or clients. Indeed, some universities and service providers have a hierarchy of levels at which researchers might reasonably use patients/clients in their research, with even masters degree students being confined to literature-based studies or research proposals for this reason. Over-researching specific populations and the workload of already overburdened ethics committees are the main reasons given.

Another important, but less explicit reason is the increasing sensitivity of service providers to potentially critical information being available to non-employees. This, they fear, might appear in the media. I myself had my 'ethical approval' for an ethnographic study withdrawn when the hospital I planned to study became the subject of media attention after a well-known 'whistleblower' (Graham Pink) published allegations in the newspapers. Secondary reasons are the waste of patients' time or worse, the possibility that patients may be harmed, upset or have their expectations raised by even interview-based studies. To return more directly to the concept of intervention as understood in the experimentalist school of thought, and with apologies to Joseph Heller, we can see a 'catch 22' situation for the researcher who would like systematically to evaluate a novel clinical intervention.

Catch 22

Imagine for a moment that I wished to test the effect of lavender oil applied during aromatherapy. If I have no evidence that such a therapy is beneficial, then surely I should do a study, preferably a randomised controlled trial, which for many provides the best kind of evidence. On the other hand, if I have no evidence that the application of lavender oil is harmless, surely such a study involves too much risk. Prashar et al. (2004) report that (in test tubes):

> *Lavender Oil (Lavandula angustifolia)... (which is) chiefly composed of linalyl acetate (51%) and linalool (35%), is considered to be one of the mildest of known plant essential oils and has a history in wound healing. Concerns are building about the potential for irritant or allergenic skin reactions with the use of lavender oil. This study has demonstrated that lavender oil is cytotoxic to human skin cells in vitro (endothelial cells and fibroblasts) at a concentration of 0.25% (v/v) in all cell types tested.*

> (Prashar 2004)

To be fair to lavender oil, Prashar et al. argue that these damaging effects are possibly the source of any therapeutic effects. The point is that in order to undertake or approve a study such as this, an investigator or an ethics committee drawing on the experimentalist view would reasonably require evidence that potential benefits exist and that harms, if any, are calculable, are in proportion to likely benefits and can be rapidly detected and dealt with. To put this another way, in order to have an ethical foundation for undertaking an intervention, we need both to have good evidence that the intervention is likely to be beneficial, and that any harms are greatly outweighed by these benefits.

In the real world, this presents as a 'catch 22', because until studies of this type are done to provide such evidence, such studies will not be justifiable from this experimental or hygienic perspective. In the real world, however, even experimental research is messier than this, and we need to cope with less certainty in some situations.

Take as an example a study in which newly diagnosed patients with leukaemia undergoing radiation and chemotherapy in an isolation unit were offered an intervention of aromatherapy massage as a diversionary measure and to reduce stress (Stringer 2005). In this study, patients were randomised either to be offered the massage intervention on a body site chosen by them, or to receive usual care. Previously, the direct evidence for benefit of such a therapy for this group of patients did not exist. This would seem like a good reason to do the study to confirm or refute the theory that such therapy is useful in some way.

On the other hand, we have no evidence that it is not harmful. One of the massage oils to be used is lavender, which as we have seen may have some irritant or allergenic properties. Even worse, in a leukaemia unit the point of isolation is to reduce the risk of life-threatening infection during the period of profound immuno-suppression. With no evidence to the contrary (in fact no evidence at all) we must assume that there is a risk in allowing the therapist into the isolation unit, with the consequent increase in potential for cross infection. Indeed, the nurse therapist/researcher in this particular study also had to collect central venous blood from research participants to test for serum cortisol levels. This also is not completely free of the risk, for example serious blood-borne infection (Eggiman et al. 2004). A particular dilemma was present for the control group, who faced some of these risks without even the possible benefit of the massage intervention itself, an issue discussed reflexively and in some detail by Stringer in her thesis (Stringer 2005).

To summarise, all novel interventions are potentially harmful and harms must be avoided where possible for both ethical and financial reasons. On this view the trial of untried interventions is difficult or impossible. On the other hand, it also seems logical that the trial of previously well-tested interventions is unnecessary. Fortunately, RECs do not necessarily follow this remorseless logic, and relatively untried interventions can be cautiously evaluated, as Stringer shows.

As I have argued, experiments of novel interventions, unless reaching the resources and rigour amenable to large multinational corporations, can be difficult to justify. As a nurse myself, it concerns me that partly for these reasons, nurses in particular among other health professionals have become distanced from experimental methods because qualitative research has been seen as somehow more relevant to the concerns of a caring, rather than a treatment-focused, occupation. I regularly ask groups of nurses to specify an experiment, done by a nurse with patients, which had findings they regularly use in their practice. On the rare occasions that anyone has a study in mind it is usually Jenny Boore's celebrated *Prescription for recovery* (1978). Avoiding the problems of studying a completely novel intervention for which no evidence existed, Boore reviewed a good deal of evidence that giving information to patients before threatening events was likely to be beneficial, and little in the way of harms could be found (see Chapter 6).

Relevant theories of stress and adaptation and the role of information in reducing stress were well known, so Boore undertook to test this theory in a novel context, with routine surgery patients in hospital wards in South Manchester. She compared 20 minutes' general chat with focussed teaching about breathing, exercises and other aspects of 'successful post-operative recovery'. This could only have been justified on grounds of replication with modification of a nursing intervention in which she had a good deal of confidence already. If Boore had been intervening in a way which was more controversial and less obviously sensible we may wonder whether a modern ethics committee (which she did not face as such) would have approved such a study. Particularly problematic would be the placebo intervention of general chat to which the control group was exposed. The study depended for its success on this having no comparable therapeutic value. In other words the chief moral difficulties were the waste of patients' time at best and the deliberate withholding of an intervention thought to be of value (the teaching and information). These proved problematic. Boore concedes that, as with Stringer 25 years later, the research assistants were troubled by failing to provide the teaching and information intervention to the control group, but for the most part they satisfied the research protocol.

The bottom line

This argument can be developed further. To illustrate why intervention may be less welcome in positivist research I will cite other examples. In an early British study, which I mention briefly in Chapter 6, Jones (1975) (who was a nurse) observed the feeding of unconscious neurosurgical patients and concluded that this was unsystematic and nutritionally ill-founded. His most famous observation was that a nurse poured apparently scalding hot fluid down a naso-gastric tube and he felt it would have compromised his place as a scientist to have intervened to prevent this. Jones was working at the very birth of substantial nursing research in the UK and perhaps he may be forgiven. Indeed, as with Boore (1978) and Oakley (1990), the research team found it difficult to avoid intervention altogether. In one case they felt they had to intervene to prevent harm to a very ill patient.

Although he allowed boiling water to be syringed down an nasogastric tube, which seems inexcusable through today's eyes, Jones (1975, p. 31) admits to advising a nurse who had been using endotracheal suction for *8 minutes* that this might be the cause of the patient's hypoxia and cyanosis, and that a rest might be in order.

Clearly, even then, Jones and his assistant were struggling with dilemmas and doing their best to intervene minimally in ways that would protect the 'science' of their study. They were unconsciously developing a 'bottom line' of harmful or substandard care below which even they could not go without saying or doing something. Sadly, theirs was pretty low, but even now we must not underestimate the difficulty of identifying where we should draw this line since the nature of the incidents we might discover in practice is almost always unknown (Johnson 2004).

It is quite clear that from time to time researchers have to find a path between the role of objective researcher and caring health professional. Kate Seers' (1989) aim was to collect data on the management of pain in hospital wards. To this end she asked patients how much pain they had and then waited to see whether analgesia provided by nursing staff met patients' perceived needs. Seers admitted that at no point did she plan to improve those patients' chances of getting analgesia by telling ward staff about their pain. Such an intervention in ward routine would have compromised the study by introducing her intervention as a confounding variable.

This approach, whilst scientifically sound, leaves open the question of whether a nurse (or anyone) should leave pain and suffering unreported, even for a short time. Seers certainly adheres to the principle of 'first do no harm' since there is no direct intervention attributable to her which might be harmful. In other words, no harm came to patients in the study which would not have been present otherwise. However, patients did experience pain, in some cases severe, which she observed and documented for research purposes, and which could have been ameliorated more quickly had it been reported to nursing staff.

Seers' position here is quite usual and is not necessarily unethical. It all depends on your point of view. Nothing happened to patients that would not have happened otherwise. No action of hers *caused* any suffering, but this is to take a rather traditional view that there is a difference in moral responsibility between acting and failing to act. In moral philosophy this is called the acts and omissions doctrine. The argument is explored most popularly in relation to euthanasia, where many see the direct killing of a person as worse than allowing them to die naturally. Conversely, if the outcome is the same how are they different? I am sure that Seers' hygienic non-intervention rule would not have gone this far, that she would have failed to intervene not only to relieve pain but to save a life worth saving. However, it makes the point that what we might call the bottom line for intervention needs to be explored in each case.

In Chapter 6 I noted that Fitzsimmons and McAloon (2004) reported their concerns about the ethics of non-intervention in a study of patients awaiting coronary artery bypass surgery. Data were collected using home interviews at three points over the patients' first year on the waiting list. The study was essentially descriptive, so patients were unlikely to benefit directly from the study itself, whilst many patients experience challenging health problems during such a period of waiting. For this reason the investigators planned to provide appropriate support for these problems when detected at interview. However, as the study progressed several patients died, prompting the investigators to change their protocol towards even more direct action to ensure that apparently deteriorating patients had immediate contact with a general practitioner and the relevant cardiac surgeon or physician. A further dilemma they faced was that by these means some patients moved up the waiting list which reduced their risk of death, whilst others moved down, which may have increased theirs.

It seems to me that whilst Fitzsimmons and McAloon discuss their concerns openly and in the context of basic ethical theories, they simply acted as any skilled professionals should, in acting to reduce the risk of harm (in this case death) by enabling the patients referred to benefit from a modified risk assessment. Provided that the modification of the waiting list was on strictly clinical grounds, I can see nothing wrong with their actions. Had they, however, in the traditions of scientific objectivity, allowed these patients to deteriorate excessively, then they certainly might feel themselves culpable.

Glover (1990) and Harris (1994) make no distinction between acts and omissions in their judgement of the human responsibility to prevent harm. That is to say that a health professional is as culpable in failing to relieve pain as in causing it where none existed. This they apply to any person, but the responsibility of the health or social care professional is the greater to the degree that they may have special skill in relieving pain or any distress. In Harris's view, responsibility to relieve suffering accrues to us all in proportion to our ability to relieve it. This, arguably, goes hand in hand with being on a register of health professionals whose first principles generally include the prevention and relief of suffering.

What is important is that researchers attempting hygienic non-intervention strategies in pursuit of their pure research designs, realise that their position may not appeal to all; least of all those whose pain might have been relieved within a more flexible design.

INTERVENTION: ISSUES IN QUALITATIVE RESEARCH

Writing of a different mode of suffering, that is, the unsatisfactory and ill-informed recovery from a hysterectomy, Webb (1984) argued that to visualise research respondents as 'subjects', mere data sources without feelings or needs, is inconsistent with feminist approaches to research. In her work with women patients she found that she identified learning and health-promotion needs in many of her respondents that she would have felt guilty in not meeting to reasonable levels of professional competence. She realised that such intervention might compromise the permission she had received earlier from surgeons and the ethics committee simply to collect data by interview. Instead she decided that giving the information was a risk worth taking in meeting a more important need.

Webb took an early step towards the justification of benevo-lent, but not necessarily planned interventions in nursing research. There being a place for such exchanges between researcher and researched can be seen as health and social care professionals exercising a responsibility to meet any need that, within resources, can be met. She successfully locates this approach within a feminist perspective that, provided the reader is sympathetic to these needs taking precedence over scientific goals, seems justifi-cation enough. However, to take the view that intervention by researchers to meet needs worth meeting is an essentially and uniquely feminist thing to do is surely mistaken. All health researchers should begin to evaluate the impact of such an approach on their research design.

I have discussed researchers who used positivist methods that seem to preclude meeting day-to-day unmet client needs. Much as I would wish it otherwise, using qualitative research methods I have had similar dilemmas and have not always acted as I later would have wished. There is a long tradition within the sociological community of covert research in which direct intervention to right wrongs or relieve suffering has been avoided because it would have blown the researcher's cover. Even writing, arguably, from a feminist perspective there were elements of this approach in Lawler's celebrated study of how nurses manage 'the body' in their work and culture *Behind the Screens*:

> *I needed a good cover because I did not want people to know I was 'making observations' or 'doing research'.*
>
> (Lawler 1991, p.12)

Lawler at least discusses this as a moral dilemma and presents her justifications for us to accept or not as the case may be. She notes the problem in terms of the deprivation of research informants of informed consent to being observed. Lawler fails to recognise the other moral consequence of her covert position, that being covert renders meaningful intervention to right wrongs or relieve suffering or pain very difficult. The role is, for the professional, very frustrating and fraught with the unresolved conflict of observing practices where standards may be at great variance with one's own.

Unfortunately, this problem is not confined to, although it may be more acute in, covert research. In ethnographic work of my own I worked on a medical ward in the professional capacity of an unpaid bank staff nurse. I had an explicit research agenda, and certainly all the staff and many of the patients knew that I was collecting data. In all sorts of ways I was capable of intervention. I participated in nursing care as planned by the nurses I was working with, and where I worked with junior students I suppose that I took the lead in managing aspects of care. Using my experience I may have been able subtly to change and possibly improve the care of individuals on rare occasions where I felt I could. In general, though, as a mere invited guest, I was constantly in danger of losing my invitation. Had I had an attitude of suggesting many or radical changes to the management of care in the ward I should soon have been unwelcome.

One example may illustrate my dilemma. One man on the ward was sitting in a chair beside his bed and had a central venous (Hickman) line running into his neck. These were normally sutured into place with plaster over them so that they were fairly secure. The time was about 1pm and the ward sister was accompanying a medical ward round. Waiting for the retinue to reach the man I could not fail to notice that the line was sliding in and out of its fixation, the suture having come out. The potential dangers, such as infection (Eggiman et al. 2004) should be self-evident but I felt that introduction of infection and the pain, inconvenience and dangers of having the line re-sited were strong possibilities. The ward sister had seen it and probably so had the retinue.

My dilemma was as follows. My first instinct was to rush over and fix the line in some way. In doing so I would have invaded the sister's territory as she was in control of the situation. Rushing over would have shown me to be capable of panic; something not welcome in this relatively hi-tech area of leukaemia nursing. I would also have been implicitly questioning her judgement of the danger this man was in. I gave her a long hard look of the questioning variety and was convinced that her non-verbal behaviour said 'leave it alone', which I did. I failed to intervene to right a wrong, if that is how we should look at it. I behaved similarly in other, but perhaps less hi-tech situations, complying in large degree with the practices of my co-participants. On reflection, my best justification for not applying what I thought were at least in some respects my own standards is that I would have lost some of my 'entree' or my welcome as an uncritical participant observer.

I think it is fair to say that the greater the degree of exchange, the more give and take there is between researcher and researched, the less problematic this situation becomes. Any new bank staff nurse who was not a researcher (or indeed a student) might have felt as I did, not wanting to offend or question the clinical judgement of the experienced ward sister in that delicate early period of negotiating one's acceptance as a member of the team. With truly participant observation in nursing, a genuine contribution to ward work, especially 'dirty work' such as empty-ing commodes and mopping up spilled breakfasts, eventually earns some credibility that is denied the less participant or hygienic observer. This credibility makes contributing to decisions about care easier as time goes on, but the invited status is always present and the researcher–respondent relationship remains fragile. Interventions to prevent harms or raise standards need to be carefully considered in this context, which is not to say that such intervention should be avoided when necessary.

My overall point is that the ethnographer may not really hold a much stronger position in terms of intervening systematically to provide better pain relief, or anything else, than the experimentalist. Indeed, to intervene systematically may, even for the qualitative researcher, change the nature of the research environment in such a way as to raise questions about the credibility of the research as a description of an extant culture. It would have become something else, namely action research.

INTERVENTION AND ACTION RESEARCH

Many of these problems are, if not solved, then thrown into a more constructive focus, by action research. The whole point of action research, as commonly understood, is intervention. Lathlean (1994) argues that:

> *First, action research is about taking action in the real world and a close examination of the effects of the action taken; thus it always involves intervention.*

(Lathlean 1994).

This position is developed by Hart and Bond (1995) who argue that in the empowering type of action research the intervention may not be so discrete or identifiable as in the experimental type and may take many forms. Not only this, but many of the objections to intervention highlighted above are less pertinent within the action perspective. Intervention may be agreed with, even designed by research participants. It can be planned and just as importantly systematically evaluated. The extreme experimental/hygienic view that there should be no interventions in non-medical health research still prevails. Indeed, action research, being so messy, would never appeal to the true devotee of this hygienic research perspective. Action research, though, is of many forms and can reasonably appeal both to the phenomenologist and to the quasi-experimentalist. Stringer's (2005) study of a massage intervention and stress reduction in cancer patients is, arguably, a very structured form of action research. Certainly, to evaluate similar interventions by health professionals in day-to-day practice and in consultation with them would conform to Hart and Bond's (1995) typology of experimental action research drawing upon concepts like controlled outcomes and looking for causal processes.

To do such work within even the experimental (largely structured) action perspective allows for modifications, adaptations and, if necessary, less systematically planned interventions to meet client needs. Stringer admits in her reflexive commentary to feeling concern that control patients were giving time and blood, and accepting modest risk for no personal benefit. To this end she concedes that she usurped her own protocol and intervened with some guided imagery with some patients. Her thesis is the better for this honesty, in contrast to the artificially clean reports of some investigators.

At the empowering end of Hart and Bond's typology of action research approaches, there is even greater flexibility, within a framework of involvement of staff and clients, for the flexible response of individuals to intervene to improve care wherever this is possible. Clearly, as Webb (1984) has argued, such an approach sits well with feminist, emancipatory or user-involvement methodology. Researchers need not feel that they are impartial observers of pain and suffering, that they are 'ripping off' their respondents to get their degree or their publications.

It is important to acknowledge the place of feminist thought, both in methodology and in ethics, in developing this view. I am sure, however, that within a framework of humanistic research, a similar position must be taken. This is one in which empowerment, the raising of consciousness, negotiated and thoroughly evaluated interventions potentially of benefit to all are possible. Where interventions are disadvantageous they may be modified or stopped in consultation with participants.

INTERVENTION: THEORETICAL ISSUES

Popular ethical theory may suffer from a certain redundancy in the context of wider discussion of intervention by health researchers. In common with the 'hygienic' or experimentalist perspective in research, much moral theory relies on interventions and their consequences being predictable. The consequentialist can give an opinion that Boore's (1978) study, though half the participants got no useful teaching, was ethically justified in terms of the improved teaching and communication received by generations of subsequent patients. Such a decision was possible in advance, since Boore presumably undertook to disseminate her findings and has, of course, done this. Seers' (1989) study might have a similar utilitarian justification for her failure to intervene to relieve known pain. To have compromised the data by changing the circumstances would have rendered the study invalid and less generalisable. Thus, future patients in similar circumstances would not be likely to benefit from the hard-won conclusions drawn.

For reasons not entirely clear, researchers and health and social care professionals more generally do not usually articulate appeals to consequential ethics in justifying their behaviour. Rather, duty-based ethics prevail, at least in the rhetoric of most codes of conduct, with human rights to autonomy, confidentiality, informed consent, etc., being prominent (Gallagher & Boyd 1991, NMC 2004).

Despite this, the justification of potentially uncomfortable or even harmful procedures is elsewhere most usually advanced in utilitarian terms of benefits to future patients. An essential difficulty with these consequential justifications is the need to have some ability to predict the consequences of intervention with a degree of certainty that may render the trial obsolete. That is to say that once we know enough to be certain of safety, we will know enough not to repeat the trial.

I find planned intervention of the clinical trial variety quite hard to fit into any duty-based code. In such views the first duty is to the patient being cared for at the present (NMC 2004), so interventions (or their absence) as an aspect of research of benefit to future clients are hard to justify. Where there is a distinct possibility that the intervention may be of benefit to the participant then duty-based ethics would support it, but only where the professional would have had a duty to provide it anyway. If there is a control (no intervention) in the trial we return to our duty to provide useful care wherever and whenever it can be resourced, which makes the use of controls problematic.

As I make clear in Chapter 3, ethical frameworks vary and each has its uses. Health care ethics textbooks continue to appeal primarily, and in some cases exclusively, to the arguably patriarchal perspectives of utility and duty. Discussions depend upon clarity, prediction of consequences, and generalisability of principles from one situation to another, essentially also the tenets of logical positivism (see for example Beauchamp & Childress 2001 and their many imitators). Although it may be important to be aware of such viewpoints, feminist thinkers have made advances insufficiently recognised by most textbook writers. I am not saying that feminists are uniquely fitted to address the moral problems presented by intervention in research. Indeed, much of the theoretical background to modern emancipatory feminist thought was originally coined by men such as Marx, Mill, Habermas and Polanyi. What is important is that feminist thought has encompassed the personal, the reflexive, the contextual and the political factors that come to bear on moral decisions in research much more effectively than those nurses working within a more traditional perspective of positivism or ethnography.

Williams (1991) has suggested that ethics has been presented traditionally as thinking in 'either/or' terms. Discussion has centred on whether to intervene or not according to well established principles. So far I, too, have addressed this issue in similar terms. Williams takes our thinking forward in a way that I suggest researchers (not just women) can identify with. First, she makes the point that role boundaries are never as clear in life as they are in research reports or ethical case studies. We bring to the research encounter ourselves as professionals, as researchers, as people in the wider world, and as women or men. It is naïve to imagine that such facts of social context do not and should not impinge upon our decisions about research activity, or anything else. In particular, Williams identifies the meaning of relationships as crucial in the interplay of factors that are part of the research act and decisions therein. This aspect of her paper, perhaps more than any other, shares perspective with other key contributions to the feminist ethics literature (Edwards & Mauthner 2002) upon which we can all draw. Williams' thesis is that there is a situational logic to ethical practice that is nowhere evident in prominent textbook accounts of either research or ethics.

Williams does not pretend that such a situational position in thinking about ethics makes principles like 'I am committed to practice in such a way as not to hurt those I encounter' (p. 66) irrelevant. She is, however, concerned to identify such principles as problematic, that is they are not free of the contradictions and difficulties of everyday practice.

Clearly such a position creates a framework within which practising researchers can confront the various forms of intervention in research (or its avoidance) in a more constructive way than by obeying rules. Ethical behaviour is seen as negotiated from day to day given the social reality of the situation. Relationships, power and roles are investigated and discussed in resolution of situations as they arise, with principles like 'first do no harm' having an important, but not exclusive part to play in deciding care and research strategy. Adherents to rule-based ethical perspectives and protocols will be quick to see what may be dangers in such a contextual approach. Codes of conduct and rules aimed at discouraging interventionist research styles grew, arguably, out of experiences of wilful abuse of patients' rights both to informed consent and not to be harmed in various contexts, not least Nazi Germany. Whatever the rules, human conduct depends very much on the qualities of the people concerned and the context within which they are brought to act. Surely an ethical approach that takes these seriously into account and raises them to awareness has much to offer.

CONCLUSION

In this chapter I have argued that hygienic or experimentalist conceptions of research are reducing the potential for health and social care professionals to engage directly in work of real relevance to practice. Despite their beneficent remit, RECs and governance neurosis have added to these concerns. The pressures are to do research that avoids contact with clients and especially avoids intervention in their lives. Perhaps paradoxically, I have argued that in some cases the hygienic perspective has allowed healthcare professionals to collect data from patients where, as nurses and as people, they should have been empowered to intervene, for example to relieve pain or maintain standards. Instead, because of their hygienic research design, they felt that they should not. The overall point remains valid, that hygienic research avoids intervention with clients and therefore distances itself from useful application.

I suggest that qualitative researchers, with their emphasis on meanings and how people feel might have room for complacency that they, at least, have people at heart in their research. On the contrary, many qualitative studies are essentially hygienic in nature, that is, they avoid too much direct contact with real people, especially 'messy' people like service users, patients or clients. In particular, intervention in care as an aspect of the research process that should be explicit is rendered problematic, and therefore to be avoided. I note that even when the design is explicitly participative, the degree of intervention negotiable in any context is variable. It depends on the social skills and tact of the researcher and the extent to which they are seen as 'natives' or prepared to offer hard physical and emotional labour in return for the right both to data and to offer constructive criticism of participants in the research process. I myself have felt unresolved conflict in both intervening and failing to intervene as a patient advocate in certain circumstances where patient care or basic standards were under threat.

During the execution of a substantial ethnographic project (Johnson 1997) I became troubled by what could be seen as the fundamental ethical flaw. That is (to paraphrase Karabel & Halsey 1977) a troubled world needs change, not mere understanding. I was able to help people in small ways but had neither mandate nor real mechanism for substantial change. I argue that action research, despite its problematic nature, contains the potential to remedy both of these omissions. Properly negotiated and in consultation with participants in the setting, useful interventions can be planned and executed that have the mandate of those present and are logistically sensible. Ethics committees and supervisory bodies for research need to recognise this and adopt a more facilitative approach to this form of interactive action research than I perceive is presently the case.

I have suggested that utilitarianism and duty-based ethics can offer some justifications for the strategies that researchers employ when interventions or their avoidance can be predicted and planned for (i.e. hygienic). Despite my self-evident bias toward consequential approaches, I recognise that these frameworks are, however, ineffective in resolving the ethical turmoil of much real-world research that is messy. Instead, I note the potential of contextual or relational ethics in which much progress has been made by feminist thinkers such as Williams (1991).

It can be argued that men are liable to encroach upon feminist thinking to make it relevant to their own needs, and in doing so sanitise it of its radicalism, its inherent threat to the dominant position of men, and their own epistemology and ethical perspectives. Of course, here I am vulnerable to such a criticism. On the other hand I can appeal to feminist ethics in its sense of relativism and relevance to context, to argue that a messy ethics is necessary for a messy context for research such as health and social care. I suggest that it may be constructive to call this approach, available to both sexes, a humanistic one.

REFERENCES

Beauchamp TL, Childress JF (2001) Principles of biomedical ethics. Oxford University Press, Oxford.

Boore JRP (1978) Prescription for recovery. Royal College of Nursing, London.

Bradby MB (1990) Status passage into nursing: undertaking nursing care. Journal of Advanced Nursing 15, 1363–1369.

Edwards R, Mauthner M (2002) Ethics and feminist research: theory and practice. In: Mauthner M, Birch M, Jessop J, Miller T (eds) Ethics in qualitative research. Sage, London.

Eggiman P, Sax H, Pittet D (2004) Catheter–related infections. Microbes and infection 6, 1033–1042

Fitzsimmons D, McAloon T (2004) The ethics of non–intervention in a study of patients awaiting coronary artery bypass surgery. Journal of Advanced Nursing 46(4), 395–402.

Gallagher U, Boyd KM (1991) Teaching and learning nursing ethics. Scutari, Harrow.

Glover J (1990) Causing death and saving lives. Penguin, Harmondsworth.

Harris J (1994) The value of life: an introduction to medical ethics. Routledge, London.

Hart E, Bond M (1985) Action research for health and social care: a guide to practice. Open University Press, Buckingham.

Johnson M (1997) Nursing power and social judgement. Ashgate. Aldershot.

Johnson M (2004) Real world ethics and nursing research. NT Research 9(4), 251–261.

Jones D (1975) Food for thought. Royal College of Nursing, London.

Karabel J, Halsey AH (Eds) (1977) Power and ideology in education. Oxford University Press, New York.

Kratz C (ed.) (1979) The nursing process. Baillière Tindall, London.

Lathlean J (1994) Choosing an appropriate methodology. In: Buckledee J, McMahon R (eds) The research experience in nursing. Chapman and Hall, London.

Lawler J (1991) Behind the screens: Nursing, somology, and the problem of the body. Churchill Livingstone, Melbourne.

Nursing and Midwifery Council (2004) The NMC Code of Conduct: Standards for conduct, performance and ethics. NMC . London

Prashar A, Locke IC, Evans CS (2004) Cytotoxicity of lavender oil and its major components to human skin cells. Cell Proliferation. 37(3), 221–229.

Seers K (1989) Patients' perceptions of pain. In: Wilson–Barnett J, Robinson S (eds) Directions in nursing research. Scutari, Harrow.

Street AF (1992) Inside nursing: a critical ethnography of clinical nursing practice. State University of New York Press, New York.

Webb C (1984) Feminist methodology in nursing research. Journal of Advanced Nursing 9(3), 249–256.

Williams A (1991) Practical ethics: interpretive processes in an ethnography of nursing. In: Aldridge J, Griffiths V, Williams A (eds) Rethinking: feminist research processes reconsidered. Feminist Praxis, Monograph 33.

12 Dissemination: ethics and aesthetics

Martin Johnson

INTRODUCTION

Writing journal articles and preparing conference presentations might seem straightforward. We hope and believe that all the ethical issues were planned for and addressed during the study itself. In fact, some of the greatest dilemmas and challenges can come at the dissemination stage of a project, and can become quite haunting. Reputations can be made and ruined at this point. For example, academic journals frequently have 'retractions' of papers that have been published because of academic fraud, plagiarism or untrue claims having been made. Sometimes these arise from genuine inexperience of the authors, sometimes from a deliberate attempt to gain credit inappropriately. Contentious issues include the attribution of authorship, conflicts of interest and the degree to which institutional and individual anonymity are helpful or necessary.

In the wider context of grave research misconduct noted in Chapter 3 a number of the issues I will discuss here are at differing points on a continuum from 'ethics' to 'aesthetics' (or good and bad taste). Nevertheless, the high standards expected of professional researchers demand their proper consideration.

THE OBLIGATIONS TO DISSEMINATE

On the whole the social care, allied health and nursing professions, given their relatively new position in the academic hierarchy, undertake excellent research. On the other hand, even in the more established scientific disciplines only relatively rarely have major discoveries been made on which lifetime reputations are established. I await anything comparable to the elucidation of the double helix of DNA.

Moreover, relatively little work has clear patent or commercial implications. For these reasons, there would seem to be little to fear from immediate dissemination of study outcomes, since other researchers ought to be unlikely to 'steal' commercially very lucrative ideas. Despite this, health researchers can be very protective of their work, sometimes to the extent that it is never published in any form.

Mann (2002) notes that research ethics committees (RECs) have received just criticism for not ensuring that the results of research they approve are properly published. Clearly, he sees that part of the 'ethical contract' with research participants and other stakeholders is that the outcomes, positive, negative or equivocal, should be properly disseminated. Indeed, it is widely held in science that results, however important, do not exist until they have been published and subjected to the scrutiny of critical peer review.

Writing particularly of clinical trials, Mann (2002) argues that a number of obligations are placed on researchers (Box 12.1).

Mann continues that approval of a study presupposes that the study has a value to society that can usually only be realised through public dissemination of outcomes. He further suggests that where research participants are altruistically involved in studies of no direct benefit to themselves (non-therapeutic), the wider benefits for others are most likely to be achieved through proper dissemination. Respondents ought to be able to discover the outcomes of studies in which they were involved and the sharing of new knowledge seems to be a reasonable moral imperative of any socially conscious science. By such means, science, in general, moves forward by enabling critical scrutiny of published

---

Box 12.1 Obligations for public dissemination of trial results (Mann 2002)

- The ethical requirement of social value presupposes results' dissemination
- Inclusion of non-therapeutic research components must be justified by acquisition of valuable knowledge
- Dissemination is necessary for production of credible and relevant systematic reviews and meta-analyses
- Public dissemination recognises the altruistic motivation of patients who agree to participate
- Participants are entitled to know results of research in which they were enrolled
- Dissemination conforms with codes of ethical conduct about sharing new knowledge with colleagues

results and the synthesis of best policy and practice through systematic reviews and meta-analyses.

Despite these good intentions, it is clear that a good deal of rivalry can exist between teams and individuals. The competitive nature of funding allocation and of promotion prospects can mean that researchers feel less inclined to share ideas than they might. On the other hand, both funds and promotion depend largely on publication records, so a sensible balance has to be struck. If secrecy is necessary, this should only be for a short time.

WHERE AND WHAT TYPE OF OUTPUT?
Conferences

The dissemination of research output can take many forms. Often the first medium of choice is one or more conference papers. Researchers will submit short abstracts of their work for selection, if suitable, by conference planning committees. This can be as much as 9 months before the occasion, which can present a dilemma. Should one send an abstract about work that, though incomplete, is expected to be finished by the conference date?

It is unwise to submit any abstract that makes claims that cannot be justified or that describes work yet to be completed *as if* it has been finished. On the other hand, an abstract can certainly describe a work in progress provided this is clear to the selection committee. Conferences are meant to be opportunities to test ideas and initial results against a constructively critical audience, and so need not always involve the 'finished product'. They can also become an opportunity to meet up with colleagues, others interested in your specialist area, and develop your 'network'. To return to the moral imperative to disseminate, it is easy to assume that conference papers are all-important, and they certainly have a worthwhile function. However, in order properly to satisfy the imperative to report work, and to ensure that work is permanently available in the public domain, written dissemination is essential. Although the advent of PowerPoint™ has meant that a conference presentation can be delivered from just a few screen slides with bullet points and pictures, it is good practice also to develop conference papers in written form to a level and standard that could easily become a journal article or book chapter once you have some feedback.

Journals and books

Callaham (2003) identifies the editorial policy of a leading medical journal in respect of the ethics of scientific publication. I will draw on this adding other aspects and examples. In the health-related fields a very large number of journals exist in which projects can be published, and many claim to be 'peer reviewed'. Despite this claim, there are considerable differences in the rigour applied in review and selection by different journals, and working out the popularity and 'academic prestige' of journals comes as much from experience as from 'impact factor' ratings. If there is a moral imperative to disseminate at all, logically this would seem to be the more satisfied the greater the readership of the journal. In this case, publishing in *Professional Social Work, Nursing Times* or *Nursing Standard* might reach many tens of thousands of readers, whilst many of the 'academic' journals, have a circulation of just hundreds, many of which will be libraries. Electronic access means that, through university and health service libraries, wide dissemination can occur, but mainly to those already interested enough in the topic to be searching electronic databases. It may then be wise to publish papers with these different audiences in mind, but taking care not to duplicate material unnecessarily.

DECIDING AUTHORSHIP

When more than one person is involved in a project it is important to decide who will be attributed as authors and whose contribution will be noted in some other way, such as with an acknowledgement at the end of the paper.

Hamilton and Clare (2003) argue that:

> *Authorship means that the individuals listed as having written the text take full accountability for it and rest their reputations on its truthfulness and accuracy.*
>
> (Hamilton and Clare 2003)

Developing this theme, Callaham (2003) makes the point that conceptions and traditions of 'authorship' vary between disciplines, but that it should imply:

> *...a significant intellectual contribution to the work and some role in writing the manuscript...*
>
> (Callaham 2003)

However, Callaham (2003) notes that given the variation in roles that can occur, colleagues should decide early in the research and writing process who will be authors and in what sequence. Hamilton and Clare (2003) argue that not everyone who contributes to a research project qualifies as an author, suggesting that authorship relates more to the intellectual contribution to the project rather than to the practical implementation of it. This can mean that recruitment of research subjects and the collection of data, even though significant tasks, may not qualify the individual as an author. Increasingly, some journals require a clear listing of specific roles and contributions to the project prior to publication. Certainly, as Callaham (2003) points out, it is becoming unacceptable to list 'honorary authors' by virtue of a person's power or prestige.

Conventions of the order of listing also vary. Sometimes the principal applicant for the funding or senior researcher, irrespective of the amount of work done, will expect to be first author. Hamilton and Clare (2003) refer to Nativio's (1997) recommendation that the first person listed should have made the most significant contribution, and note that generally after this the order is either alphabetical or in order of the size of the contribution.

Whether or not academic research supervisors should qualify for authorship is also slightly contentious. Many supervisors provide guidance of such depth, quality and detail that it is hard to argue that their work should not be seen as germane to the project in hand. Supervising a PhD, for example, can mean detailed reading, re-reading and annotation of manuscripts that, together with tutorials typically over a period of 4 or 5 years, can add up to hundreds of hours of work. This is time that could otherwise have been spent on the supervisor's own research. On the other hand, a PhD is by definition meant to be original work by the candidate.

Clearly it would be irregular to attribute authorship of the thesis itself to any other than the candidate. Logically, this should also apply to any publications arising from the work, but in recognition of the supervisor's contribution it has become customary in some departments to allow co-authorship of one or more of the outputs immediately arising from the work.

Given the fashion for larger supervision teams of two or three people, such arrangements should be agreed upon in advance, and should probably only apply to the supervisors who actually have done a large share of the detailed supervision. Technical help in information retrieval or of a statistical nature also may vary in its qualification for authorship. It will depend on the degree of time and effort expended and the degree to which the study could have been completed without this input. If statistical or other technical advice is vital to success of the proposal, of the project and especially of meeting publication requirements it seems to me that this qualifies for authorship.

PLAGIARISM

> *Plagiarism is the use of others' published and unpublished ideas or words (or other intellectual property) without attribution or permission, and presenting them as new and original rather than derived from an existing source.*

(Callaham 2003)

The intent is to derive undue credit for work and ideas and is described by (Callaham 2003) as scientific misconduct. Vogelsang (1997) is more specific. Drawing on the *American Medical Association Manual of Style*[1] Vogelsang lists as examples of plagiarism:

- Direct verbatim lifting of passages
- Rewording ideas from the original in the purported author's own style
- Paraphrasing the original work without attribution
- Noting the original source of only some of what is borrowed.

Whilst she offers no excuses for plagiarism, which she also describes as a 'major crime' punishable as theft of intellectual property, she does suggest that it is not always deliberate. She argues that more benevolent explanations include a lack of education or acculturation to the methods and procedures of research and simple failure of diligent scholarship.

Again, conventions vary for the citation of specific passages of text, but she suggests that where more than six words are quoted directly, these should be in quotation marks and a page number and reference given. Where images, drawings, figures and longer sections of published work are used, specific permission should be gained from the publisher and duly acknowledged in the new text.

Self-plagiarism

Self-plagiarism is the repeated use of one's own work in different publications. At first this might seem unproblematic: how does one steal one's own work? Whilst illustrating that this has its problems, Broome (2004) demonstrates that 'use of part of one's own previously copyrighted work, such as sections of a review of the literature, or descriptions of design and methods sections in a study' (p. 273) can be difficult to avoid. It is appropriate to try to reach different types of reader with differently targeted outputs,

---

[1] Which she names but does not directly reference

but where it is necessary to explain routine aspects like methods and important results, these are bound to involve some repetition.

The issue seems to be the degree to which an individual uses and re-uses one piece of work, with only slight modification, or essentially reporting the same facts, in many different locations (salami-slicing). Satisfying the need to reach many audiences, from patients, to clinicians, to other researchers, might allow for at least three broadly similar papers, one in a 'professional journal', one in an 'academic journal' and one as a simple factual report, executive summary, leaflet, or web-page.

Where practical, care should be taken to acknowledge the other forms of output in each case, and as little use as possible should be made of the same precise text. Where virtually the same paper is to be published more than once, which can be done on a planned basis, the publisher's permission should certainly be sought.

Occasionally, having produced a thesis or report, a researcher will have published several papers during the process. It is not uncommon then for the edited thesis itself to be published in book or monograph form. In such cases again, clear reference should be made to previously published sections, obtaining publishers' permission (not often withheld) to repeat any large sections of text, diagrams or figures.

DEALING WITH EDITORS

Once authors have decided their contribution and its acknowledgment and a paper has been planned or drafted, the team will then choose a form of written output for their first publication on the project. In funded work this might be a report published by the sponsor or department in which the work was done. This is referred to as 'grey literature', and though quite possibly rigorously assessed, may not be considered to have undergone the critical peer review and scrutiny of an academic journal.

Many journals accept only a fraction of the papers submitted to them, and the period in which this decision is made can be lengthy (often several months). Good sense would therefore suggest sending it to several journals to increase the chances of success. However, publishing etiquette demands that authors send any particular paper to *just one journal at a time* (Hamilton 2003). This rule may seem to favour publishers and editors over authors in what could otherwise be described as a free market for research papers. However, peer reviewers are invariably unpaid for the several hours' work they may give to refereeing a paper, and academic journals, because their subscription base is small and their advertising revenue is low, usually run on quite low budgets. If all academics routinely submitted their papers to several unsuspecting journals the system would break down and, if accepted in several publications, copyright would be infringed.

CONFLICTS OF INTEREST

Some journals now expect a declaration by the principal author that no conflicts of interest exist in relation to the publication. This can mean a number of things. For example, results of research funded by a commercial sponsor might possibly appear to favour the products of that company. Governments and other organisational sponsors also are not above encouraging the publication of results they like and discouraging it when the results do not support their policies. As Hamilton (2003) suggests, the *perception* of a conflict of interest can be as damaging as an actual one.

Simply studying one's own organisation (Williamson 2003), whilst a popular approach to learning about research and providing locally relevant outcomes, can represent a significant conflict of interest. Managers might be keen to hear of (and see published) results that show the institution in a good light. In today's climate of league tables, star ratings and competition, they may be less keen to see critical outcomes published. Investigators doing 'action research' within their own organisation need to be aware of these political and managerial constraints.

Other conflicts of interest might come into play in the role of editor or reviewer of a manuscript. Callaham (2003) suggests that even attracting lecture fees or consultancy, and certainly strong academic relationships, such as examining or supervision, can all have a bearing on objectivity in the review process. The reviewer may already hold a favourable, or unfavourable, impression of a particular author or team. They may even be related, or have a close friendship with the author. Strictly speaking, most journals send out papers to reviewers 'blinded', that is with the name and other identifying marks removed. Several factors confound this blinding process, however. First, the author may be undertaking a prominent, perhaps funded piece of work, so that most informed referees would know who was involved. Second, an author publishing several different papers about the same project will eventually become known. Third, authors may refer appropriately to their own work which, unless excluded from the references until later makes identification of the author likely. Finally, some projects are local in nature and, having perhaps agreed that institutions need not be anonymous, key stakeholders may be identifiable.

Whilst rigour and quality of articles is uppermost in the editor's mind in deciding to accept a paper, given the competition for space, other considerations can come into play. Editors themselves often examine papers without any blinding process. For many practical reasons they need to know the author details. Editors have some role in avoiding both deliberate and naive plagiarism or they may need to balance their journal editorially with papers reflecting diverse international origins. Sometimes editors need to guide authors who seem to be 'salami slicing'. They may be attempting to publish more than a reasonable number of papers from one project, even if in a technical sense, they do not constitute self-plagiarism since they are on slightly different aspects.

Whilst editors are accountable to their editorial boards and ultimately their publishers, there is, arguably, room for a lack of objectivity or even discrimination in their editorial policy. Certainly they act as 'gatekeepers' encouraging certain styles, content and approaches and discouraging others. If these are technical aspects, such as whether work is written in the first or third person or is qualitative or quantitative, then these can be debated and resolved. Of greater concern is the possibility for sexism (Cotterill & Letherby 2005), institutional racism (Gunaratnam 2003) or, as publications become more international, xenophobia.

OPEN ACCESS PUBLISHING

In traditional academic publishing in paper-based journals it is interesting that most of the hard work is done for free. The authors submit work without payment and unpaid referees review, annotate, advise on and assist in editing articles. Editors are commonly paid, but most would agree at a very modest hourly rate given their experience and position. Against these disadvantages, there are clear benefits to publication. A mixture of altruism, the moral imperative to publish and personal or institutional ambition motivate these people to produce intellectual property that is then signed over to a publisher. The publisher has considerable costs in a range of editorial, production, marketing and supply processes. These must be offset against the income from personal or institutional subscriptions, although the advent of electronic publication is modifying these in important respects. Access to such journals is available only to those who subscribe personally, or those who are students or work in institutions that have paid subscriptions.

Open-access publishing works on a different model. The director and publisher of BioMedCentral (Velterop 2004) makes a strong case that in the interests of open access to science, especially to the developing world, a different publishing model should be adopted. Generally, on this model the authors, their employers or sponsors pay for a paper to be considered for publication (Gass 2005). 'Author or sponsor pays' is not so strange. Most researchers already accept this model for conference attendance, paying many hundreds of pounds, when the benefits of attendance are much less permanent than an article. On the open access model, once published, the paper is made available though the World Wide Web free to those with access to an Internet connection. In some cases, paper versions of the journal can still be purchased as an extra.

From the point of view of a moral imperative to disseminate as widely as possible and on an international scale, this model has some appeal. Even in a well-resourced department of a university research can be very frustrating when the journals accessed are not available without further, sometimes considerable, payment. Velterop argues that for researchers:

> *...full access to the fruits of earlier research efforts is of vital importance for any effective scientific research...*
>
> (Velterop 2004)

He notes that the traditional subscription model is no longer suitable for scientific communication because it imposes restrictions on access and usage of literature that are only lifted after payment is made. He admits that such restrictions were inevitable in the pre-World Wide Web era, but now sees a future of complete open access to science that must be in everyone's (except perhaps publishers') interests.

An argument can be made that, in common with some conferences with very large attendances, the potential for income from delegates, or in this case authors, encourages the acceptance of lower standards of paper. Velterop (2004) objects, however, that (unlike conferences) payment is for *consideration* of a paper and does not guarantee publication, just as paying for a driving test does not guarantee a licence.

It may be fair to say that open access publishing is posing a major threat to the traditional publishing model to the extent that many large publishing houses are responding in a number of ways. For example, some provide access to 'developing countries at preferential rates' and are investing some of their profits in making even the whole back-catalogue of papers electronically available under subscription. The first volume of *The Lancet* from the early 19th Century is available on www.sciencedirect.com (The Lancet 1823) but you will only have access if you or your library subscribes.

A number of health-related publications have attempted the open-access approach. For example, the *On-line Journal of Issues in Nursing* (http://www.nursingworld.org/ojin/) is based in a department at Kent State University USA. It is supported by the university and by staff and a wider circle of academics who provide copy and editorial assistance for free. Already having a range of well-known contributors to themed issues, it will be interesting to see how effective, influential and academically valued the journal becomes, and what threat, if any, such media will pose to traditional avenues of output.

HOW IMPORTANT ARE ANONYMITY AND CONFIDENTIALITY?

In preparing a research report it is commonly seen as good practice to assure research participants and organisations of their anonymity and of the confidentiality of the data collected. This can mean changing or hiding the names of both individuals and organisations. In larger studies this may be straightforward, but in small or localised studies this can be quite challenging. Sometimes, in a misplaced attempt to improve anonymity, where a particular gender is rare, individuals' genders are even changed, but this goes too far. This approach ignores the importance that we know gender has in our understanding of social roles.

Similarly, it is important to acknowledge that some styles of research, such as history, demand that individual names and roles are made clear or the text is meaningless. It is important to maintain academic integrity here, which can mean writing things that may be critical or painful for some. Provided that sound evidence is offered for interpretations and conclusions to be drawn, then the historian writes about real events in their proper context. Fortunately, there may be some protection from the elapse of time.

Many television documentaries about health care are in some ways analogous to research and contain extremely personal information about named respondents, but provided the individuals concerned give consent to the publication of these data, the programme is screened. Further thought is needed about the relative risks and benefits, and the validity of the comparison between investigative or documentary journalism and research. Nevertheless, the convention of rendering research participants and organisations anonymous in reports is probably wise in most cases. Where identities are to be revealed this should be agreed in writing in advance of any publication or report.

CONSTRUCTIVE CRITICISM

An explanation sometimes offered by those who fail to disseminate their work appropriately is the fear of criticism. To date, this fear is generally unfounded. At conferences, whilst occasionally a legitimate and penetrating question may be asked about a study, a genuine answer is almost always accepted. Researchers understand the degree of experience that the presenter seems to have, and generally reserve their more challenging questions for those with more experience. Where presenters are new and unused to the setting of a large conference, they might seek the support of colleagues and supervisors at their presentations, which can be very reassuring. On the other hand some of us are more nervous with colleagues than we are with delegates we do not know.

Before sending a work for publication the authors are wise to seek informal peer review from experienced researchers. It is remarkable how rarely new authors seek the benefit of the advice of their senior and much more experienced colleagues in this respect. This process will almost certainly reduce the level and depth of criticism that editors and reviewers can provide when they finally receive the paper. Part of this peer-review process should be focussed on the report of ethical aspects of the study. Much control of ethical standards is through informal peer scrutiny of this type, where a gentle sanction can be applied if a researcher has begun to use inappropriate approaches.

Before the work is published, it is subjected to rigorous peer review and moderated by at least one experienced editor. In by far the majority of cases, authors will be asked to make revisions to their manuscript, most of which will be reasonable. It is wise to assume that, however tedious, most of these are really necessary. From time to time, however, reviewers will have missed the point, or may even have less expertise on a particular point. In such cases the author should discuss the points with the editor and make a case that the text should remain as it is. As we have said, authors are responsible for the words written, and so they must only accept changes with which they can be comfortable.

Having argued that most work receives no serious criticism, I will argue here that it should. The allied health disciplines, nursing and social work have come only in the last few decades to full recognition as university-based academic subjects. For this reason the traditions of strong but impersonal criticism prevalent in philosophy, psychology, sociology and medicine are at an early stage of development in nursing and health-related areas. As I have noted in Chapter 6, significant criticism of the *ethical* conduct of research is minimal. Similarly, despite the skills of critical appraisal becoming common, these skills are rarely used in the analysis of published work in a detailed way. Work which does not meet specified criteria, rather than being analysed for its weaknesses, is simply discarded.

Literature reviews are all too commonly mere lists of previous work in which little or no discussion of methods, perspective or ethics takes place. Even postgraduate theses, in which there is more space for detailed critique, often cover much ground by reviewing very many papers but saying little about any (Spouse & Johnson 2002). This may be because authors feel they need to demonstrate 'wide' reading, but depth is frequently lacking. Of course, criticism must be fair, it must be based on criteria that are explicit, and it must not be personalised. In particular, if we criticise the work of others, we must ourselves learn to cope with the prospect of scrutiny of our own work. This is simply the dialectic through which knowledge is said to advance, which is surely our overall aim.

CONCLUSION

In this final chapter I have explained a number of the benefits of dissemination of research that ought to outweigh any supposed disadvantages. In the light of the implied or actual contract with research participants and other stakeholders, sponsors, employer, other researchers and society in general, I suggest that there is a strong obligation to publish. I enumerate a range of forms of output, from websites and leaflets, which might be better suited to service users, patients and clients, to conferences, journals and books. I examine a number of issues that, whilst at the margins of 'right and wrong' in terms of the label 'ethics', are important conventions in research conduct. These include deciding on authorship, avoiding conflicts of interest and plagiarism and dealing with editors.

The wider issue of the future of publishing is considered in the context of the World Wide Web and the advent of 'open-access' publishing. I conclude by making a case that with dissemination comes a duty to be open to constructive criticism both of and from others.

REFERENCES

Broome M (2004) Self-plagiarism: Oxymoron, fair use, or scientific misconduct. Nursing Outlook 52, 273–274.

Callaham M (2003) Journal policy on ethics in scientific publication. Annals of Emergency Medicine 41(1), 82–89.

Cotterill P, Letherby G (2005) Women in Higher Education: Issues and challenges. Women's Studies International Forum 28, 109–113.

Gass A (2005) Paying to free science: costs of publication as costs of research. Serials Review 31(2), 103–106.

Gunaratnam Y (2003) Researching 'race' and ethnicity: methods, knowledge and power. Sage, London.

Hamilton H (2003) Ties that bind: ethical and legal issues for writers. In: Clare J (ed.) Writing research: transforming data into text. Churchill Livingstone, Edinburgh.

Hamilton H, Clare J (2003) Key relationships for writers. In: Clare J (ed.) Writing research: transforming data into text. Churchill Livingstone, Edinburgh.

Mann H (2002) Research ethics committees and public dissemination of clinical trial results. The Lancet 359, 406.

Nativio D (1997) Guidelines for nurse authors and editors. CINAHL News Publishers' Edition 98(1).

Spouse J, Johnson M (2002) Appropriate criticism. Clinical Effectiveness in Nursing 6, 1–2.

The Lancet (1823) Extracts from the Lancet. The Lancet, Volume 1(1), 10–12.

Velterop J (2004) Open access: science publishing as science publishing should be. Serials Review 30(4), 308–309.

Vogelsang J (1997) Plagiarism – An act of stealing. Journal of PeriAnesthesia Nursing 12(6), 422–425.

Williamson TK (2003) Building the evidence base for shared governance: the Rochdale experience. In: Edmonstone J (ed.) Shared governance: making it work. Kingham Press, Chichester.

13

Research ethics in the real world: conclusions

Martin Johnson

Given that the book title includes 'research ethics' one might be forgiven for thinking that this is a book about philosophy. No author of a chapter is a philosopher in the formal understanding of the term. We don't claim to understand the subtle and not so subtle differences between the earlier and the later Wittgenstein, although we feel he had as much to offer as the fashionable but largely irrelevant Heidegger. Wittgenstein's quest for conceptual clarity and powerful logic has clearly influenced some of the major health-care ethicists of our time, such as John Harris, and we have tried to follow a similar path. We hope that our general risk–benefit approach to the book makes it useful in a way that 'codes of conduct' and absolute principles such as 'do no harm' might not.

In these concluding remarks I intend to draw attention to some underlying themes and make a plea for some funding bodies and investigators to turn their sights on examining and working towards solutions for some of the issues and problems health and social care investigators face. I mean real problems such as whether or when to intervene to right wrongs, and bureaucratic ones such as requiring honorary contracts to conduct staff surveys by questionnaire. I will try to draw out some aspects of the concept of respect for the individual that is implied in previous chapters and will ask further questions about the balance of rigour and integrity in research.

RESEARCHING RESEARCH ETHICS

It is clear that the subject of research ethics in health and social care has not been investigated sufficiently empirically. A great deal of literature, some of which we discuss in this book, debates the actual and supposed ethical issues confronting both quantitative and qualitative researchers. There are codes of conduct, guidelines and a good deal of prescriptive information about 'informed consent', confidentiality and rights and duties.

A lesser, but important body of work offers reflections on actual studies and the ethical issues and problems encountered. Studies that appeared to cross certain boundaries, such as Humphreys' (1975) *Tearoom Trade* and Milgram's (1974) *Obedience to Authority* have been reflected upon and hotly debated, with a good deal of convenient hindsight. More recently, with the rise of 'reflexivity', investigators have examined and sometimes agonised over their own moral dilemmas (Lawton 2000, Seymour et al. 2005). Others analyse the way that they have been treated by the ethics and governance bureaucracy. For example, Hannigan and Allen (2004) illustrate the differential treatment they received at the hands of two NHS Ethics Committees, noting in particular that whilst their two studies had similar methodology, the idea of studying respondents with a diagnosis of mental health problems may have provoked excessive ethics committee concerns.

Rather than analyse their personal experiences, but surely motivated by them, Howarth and Kneafsey (2004), the authors of Chapter 7, undertook a regional survey of investigators' experiences of 'research governance' in the UK health service. They found a good deal of awareness of it as such, but also that respondents felt that there was a general lack of clarity in its implementation. Many felt that despite its laudable aims, research governance as then implemented hindered even very simple and innocuous research on a number of levels. Students were discouraged from any kind of empirical work and processes still reflected the predominance of medical research designs. Their study, despite their best efforts, was funded only by a small university grant.

It would be unfair to claim that no useful work has been done. Julia Neuberger (1992) conducted a comprehensive survey by questionnaire and interview of the terms of reference, membership, work and policy issues of UK health service research ethics committees. She produced many recommendations, many of which were broadly adopted, although the more detailed monitoring of research processes, such as spot checks of consent and methods of recruitment, seem not to be current practice. Apart from a brief end-of-study report, most approval agencies take the claims of investigators, rightly or wrongly, at face value.

If we are to put research ethics on a more empirical footing, Sieber (2001) proposes a framework for the discussion of 'research on research ethics'. She argues that until the 1960s 'most scientists considered their work value free or inherently good' and that most researchers were oblivious to the ethical dimensions of their work. 'The field of research on research ethics was beyond the imagination of everyone' she continues (p. 13236). Despite a few examples, this latter view could be held true today; the range of aspects of research ethics she feels could be better studied are shown in Box 13.1.

I wholeheartedly agree. Research ethics is so complex that a book such as this merely opens a door to a world of interplay between values, methods, benefits and harms. In order to enable greater clarity for everyone, there needs to be a good deal of research, thought and discussion between people as diverse as service users, philosophers, practitioners and academics.

RESPECT FOR INDIVIDUALS

Throughout this book the authors have emphasised the importance of recognising the preferences of potential or actual research participants and paying due respect to their choices as individuals. In order to accord respect to those whom we might study in

---

Box 13.1 Research into research ethics: some topics and questions (after Sieber 2001)

- Surveys of compliance with regulations
- Study of the scientific and ethical values of researchers
- Observational studies of the nature of informed consent
- Study of the balance of risk–benefit in different types of research
- Equity audit, that is to say investigation of the degree to which subjects/respondents are treated equitably by gender, race, culture, disability, social class or other factor
- Assessment of the actual beneficial or other outcomes of studies
- Investigation of the comprehension of those supposed to have given 'informed consent'
- Under what conditions might covert or other now ethically unfashionable methods be justified?
- How might researchers deal with the paradox of privacy: that is, that in order to study privacy, dignity and respect they must be to some degree invaded?
- What are the actual risks to patient confidentiality by data storage?
- Assessment of the extent and effects of plagiarism in any or all of its forms.

research, we need to think clearly about the boundaries of membership of this elusive population; who or what must be accorded that respect, and what should be done about humans or human material at the margins of the population?

Foetal material and developing embryos present one of the most difficult areas of research on which to make convincing ethical decisions. At 14 days after fertilisation, the research embryo gains special legal (and perhaps moral) status. After these 2 weeks the new embryo can no longer be treated merely as experimental material. Always undeniably human material, differentiation from this point into tissues that will recognisably become foetus or umbilical material causes sufficient concern that from 14 days the subject of the research would inevitably be human and at least potentially a human individual. This date was decided by the UK parliament on the advice of the Warnock Committee, which could not be unanimous about when such tissue should be deemed to be irrevocably human (Warnock 1984). It was a compromise between those who felt that even a new conceptus should be experimentally inviolable, and those who would argue that true 'human' nature grew rather later, in terms of weeks or months.

Another perhaps extreme but important example of a human population that provokes difficult decisions about its use in research is that of anencephalic babies (infants born without a cerebrum). It is difficult to conceive of any interests that such babies (and later children) may hold since they have never possessed the anatomical apparatus with which to think, hold opinions, or form values. This, together with their inability to express any preference or desire on any topic provokes something of a paradox in a research world in which informed consent and prevention of harm take precedence, yet each is meaningless in this specific case.

Other groups of individuals who have lost competence permanently pose similar problems. Gelling (2004), for example, makes arguments that individuals in a persistent vegetative state ought not to be excluded from research merely because they cannot express preferences about their own lives, and similar arguments could be made about those with dementia. As ever, a balance has to be struck between allowing the population to benefit from research and avoiding undue risks of individuals being badly treated or given insufficient respect. The same is true even of the dead. The problems which arose at the Royal Liverpool Children's Hospital over inappropriate disposal of human tissue suggest that respect should be accorded to the body parts of those long dead (House of Commons 2001).

While there has been insufficient space in this book to address all of these issues in the depth that we would have liked, they remain important problems to be addressed in terms of research ethics and some may assume increasingly more importance in future.

BUREAUCRACY OR INTEGRITY?

We have explained in Chapters 7, 8 and 9 how to get ethics and governance approval and how such things are but a partial safeguard of ethical standards or, more importantly, the reduction of unnecessary harms to research participants. The bureaucracy only goes so far, however. A curriculum, however well written and approved by university committees, is only as good as the knowledge and abilities of the teachers and students who take part in it. Similarly, a research proposal depends for its execution on the skills and integrity of the investigators and participants.

The pressures to do research and to publish are great, and for some greater than others. Some researchers, for example, need to generate sufficient income from grants alone to fund their posts, and grants are most likely to be awarded to those with strong, relevant, publications. Threats to researcher integrity, and which approval procedures can do little about, come in many forms.

The world of research is competitive. One must compete for grants, journal space or the right to present at conferences, and even to be elected to membership of important committees. Even at the student level, the marking or grading of assignments and degrees can lead to students competing rather than collaborating in retrieving learning resources or key references. Additionally, in developing to more senior levels it is important to develop 'presence'. This means being known for what you do, being seen as a leading researcher in your field. Doing top-quality research may not be enough to get you noticed, so the tactics include being 'seen' at conferences, asking questions of important speakers and reminding everyone of your name and where you are from. Sometimes known as 'showboating', this can also be evident in publications. Whilst on the one hand institutions reasonably want credit for their support, sometimes work is done in an attempt to promote rather than to evaluate critically. The margins between dissemination and marketing become blurred.

The search for high impact factors (the number of times work is cited by others) can also be a driver. Certainly at least one journal currently with a high impact factor (Nursing Science Quarterly) can be fairly described as promoting the work of one person in particular; much of its content claims to 'confirm' a particular theory by Parse (Johnson 1999). In 2005 the Times Higher Education Supplement (Baty 2005) reported on a dispute between researchers at the University of Sheffield and drug manufacturers Proctor and Gamble (Box 13.2).

This case explodes the myth that medical research is wholly done by the medical researchers themselves. In some cases, the health service and university staff are merely acting, despite their research reputations, as subject recruiters and data collectors.

Box 13.2 Data row sparks research debate

An urgent debate on the responsibilities of academics when authoring research papers was demanded this week after it emerged that university researchers collaborating with a pharmaceutical company had published findings without full access to the drug trial data on which the conclusions were based. The case has highlighted a divide between academics and industry over what is considered acceptable practice when companies sponsor academics to produce joint research papers. The pharmaceutical industry argues that it is standard practice to limit academics' access to the results of their multimillion-pound drug-trial databases, but leading scientists argue that academics must have complete access to all findings for there to be genuine research partnerships. They say researchers should put their names to publications only if they have had full, unfettered access to data and can independently verify the conclusions. Documents obtained by The Times Higher reveal that research findings on Procter & Gamble Pharmaceutical's osteoporosis drug Actonel were released under the name of Sheffield University researchers despite the fact that the academics had not carried out their own independent analyses of the firm's drug trial data. The academics, from Sheffield's Bone Metabolism Research Unit, published a journal article with the incorrect declaration that 'all authors had full access to the data and analyses'. The company initially refused requests to allow the academics to carry out their own independent analyses of the data, and when one of the research team finally gained supervised access to some data, he expressed doubts about the conclusions being drawn.

Extract from report by Phil Baty. In the Times Higher Education Supplement. 25 November 2005

Whilst less-privileged researchers in the rest of the health and social care sector might at first envy the help such as given by drug companies to some medical researchers ('ghost-writers'), they might be nervous of the distance from raw data with which others are comfortable. On the secondary question of conflict of interest, no-one can doubt that drug companies have a vested interest in drawing certain conclusions about their products. As explained in Chapter 12, first or any attributed authorship, as a matter of integrity, ought to mean that the author had a serious part to play in some aspect of the study above and beyond the instrumental aspects of recruitment and routine data collection.

On December 23rd 2005 news broke that Professor Hwang Woo Suk, widely regarded as one of the world's leading experts on cloning, stepped down from his chair at the Seoul National University amid allegations by an investigating panel that he had fabricated results of human stem cell lines. His work had been published in the most prestigious of journals, *Science*. An important point is that a colleague drew attention to inconsistencies, a role that demands courage and integrity.

The discovery of actual mistakes and falsehoods is relatively rare, but, like drug errors, probably suffers from a good deal of under-reporting, and for the same reason, which is that the person responsible is also responsible for the report. Among the most celebrated British cases was that of educational psychologist Sir Cyril Burt.

Having demonstrated the high degree of heritability of intelligence in studies of twins separated at birth, Burt was accused of fabricating most of his results. This was the more embarrassing since he had been the chief advisor in the construction of education policy of the time, which was based on his theories, the segregation of pupils at age 11+ by tested 'intelligence' levels. Burt was said to have believed so strongly in his theories that he felt data to be unimportant. Supporters of Burt have argued that despite the dubious nature of his data, his results were consistent with many other studies. Rushton (2002), for example, argues that Burt was wrongly accused. The veracity of the claims and counterclaims may now be less important than the lessons we should learn. Raw data of any kind should be kept, if necessary in a suitably anonymous form, for decades, so that accusations of falsehood can be countered with data. In my view this applies to qualitative and quantitative research, and bureaucratic appeals to 'destroy data' on completion of studies are gravely mistaken.

With Burt some form of closer scrutiny and challenge ought to have been possible, but we can assume that his massive reputation got in the way, and certainly the current research management and ethics committees, even at today's standards, might have been unlikely to reveal his type of misconduct if, indeed, that is what it was.

CONCLUSION

As health and social care professionals we must accept that the approval of research projects to be undertaken will, where such projects are submitted to them, be under the control of research bureaucracy in the form of committees or individual gatekeepers. We would be foolish, however, to imagine that these measures, however rigorously applied, will protect the public from all extremely poor conduct or 'unethical' research. Many ethical problems are all but unknown until the study begins, when to all intents and purposes ethics committees have signed the work off. No amount of 'clinical governance' nor even the General Medical Council (by whom he had earlier been investigated for drug abuse) protected people from the general practitioner and multiple murderer Harold Shipman. Similarly, the professional conduct machinery of the nursing profession has sometimes failed remarkably in its duty to protect the public (by removal from the register), for example from Philip Donnelly, a prison-served convicted child abuser (Long 1992).

More important, possibly, than the ever-present bureaucracy are means to develop, maintain and scrutinise the integrity and standards of individuals and groups engaged in research. Assuming that selection is good, this will mean better education about important issues and their possible solution, and vigorous debate together with the fuller use of peer-review as considered in Chapter 9. As we have argued, these phenomena are still but in their infancy, at least in health and social care. Research ethics in many research training programmes is a lecture or a study day at best.

We have discussed the notion of respect for the individual that underlies the thinking in much of the book, but suggest that currently no particular model of this will be acceptable to all. Issues particularly at the beginning and end of life, perhaps at the margins of life, will continue to prompt concern and debate. That is to say that however logical it may be to treat specimens from the deceased as valueless, as the furore over such public scandals has demonstrated, so long as they matter to someone they must be treated with respect. At the same time, unthinking dismissal of the possibility of research on human subjects who are unable to consent (such as those in a persistent vegetative state) negates the potential for a section of society to gain from the outcomes of research. Similarly, while technological advances and research continue to outpace ethical thinking and legislation in the fields of embryology, germ cell manipulation and cloning, for example, clear thinking and objective review of risks and potential benefits to individuals and groups must supplant raw emotion and uncritical, polarised stances in the management of research activity.

In particular, we have argued that the area of research ethics is itself insufficiently investigated. Despite those who see philosophy and its specialist branch, ethics, as an armchair activity, we maintain that many of the issues could very usefully be studied by various empirical means and with great benefit to all those involved. We hope that our book will help in some way in achieving an awareness of fundamentals like respect for the individual, benefit and risk; in raising questions about previous studies and current ones; and in understanding the viewpoints that can usefully be brought to bear on problems. We offer some practical advice on getting through the bureaucracy and raise issues in the use of new Internet technologies for research. Overall, we hope that we urge researchers at all levels to recognise that in the 'real world' we need to balance rigour and integrity with transparent pragmatism.

REFERENCES

Baty P (2005) Data row sparks research debate. Times Higher Education Supplement, 25th November. http://www.thes.co.uk/current_edition/story.aspx?story_id=20262 83 (Accessed 23rd December 2005).

Gelling L (2004) Researching patients in the vegetative state: difficulties of studying this patient group. NT Research 9(1), 7–17.

Hannigan B, Allen D (2003) A tale of two studies: research governance issues arising from two ethnographic investigations into the organisation of health and social care. International Journal of Nursing Studies 40, 685–695.

House of Commons (2001) Royal Liverpool Children's Inquiry: summary and recommendations. http://www.rlcinquiry.org.uk. (Accessed 1st August 2005).

Howarth ML, Kneafsey R (2004) The impact of research governance in healthcare and higher education organisations. Journal of Advanced Nursing 49(6), 675–683.

Humphreys L (1975) The tearoom trade. Aldine, Chicago.

Johnson M (1999) Observations on positivism and pseudoscience in qualitative nursing research, Journal of Advanced Nursing 39(1), 67–73.

Lawton J (2000) The dying process: Patients' experiences of palliative care. Routledge, London.

Long T (1992) 'To protect the public and ensure justice is done': an examination of the Philip Donnelly case. Journal of Advanced Nursing 17(1), 5–9.

Milgram S (1974) Obedience to authority: an experimental view. Harper and Row, New York.

Neuberger J (1992) Ethics and health care: the role of research ethics committees in the United Kingdom. London. King's Fund Institute.

Rushton JR (2002) New evidence on Sir Cyril Burt: His 1964 Speech to the Association of Educational Psychologists. Intelligence 30(6), 555–567.

Seymour J, Payne S, Reid D, Sargeant A, Skilbeck J, Smith P (2005) Ethical and methodological issues in palliative care studies: the experiences of a research group. Journal of Research in Nursing 10(2), 169–188.

Sieber JE (2001) Research ethics: research. International Encyclopaedia of the social and behavioural sciences. 13235–13240. http://www.sciencedirect.com/science/referenceworks/008043076 7 (Accessed 23rd December 2005).

Warnock M (1984) Report of the committee of enquiry into human fertilisation and embryology. London. HMSO.

Glossary

AoIR	Association of Internet Researchers
BPS	British Psychological Society
BSA	British Sociological Association
CERES	Consumers for Ethics in Research
COREC	Central Office for Research Ethics Committees
CPHVA	Community Practitioners' and Health Visitors' Association
CRC	Co-operative Research Centres
CRDC	Central Research and Development Committee
DH	Department of Health
EEA	European Economic Area
EU	European Union
FDA	Food and Drug Administration (US)
GMC	General Medical Council
GP	General Practitioner
HPA	Health Protection Agency
IME	Institute of Medical Ethics
INVOLVE	An advisory group to support public and patient involvement in research
IP	Intellectual property
LREC	Local research ethics committee
MDA	Medical Devices Agency
MHPRA	Medicines and Healthcare Products Regulatory Agency

MRC	Medical Research Council
MREC	Multi-centre research ethics committee
NCCSDO	National Co-ordinating Centre for NHS Service Delivery and Organisation
NHS	National Health Service
NHSE	National Health Service Executive
NMC	Nursing and Midwifery Council
OREC	Office for Research Ethics Committees
PCT	Primary Care Trust
PICTF	Pharmaceutical Industry Competitiveness Task Force
R&D	Research and development
RCM	Royal College of Midwives
RCN	Royal College of Nursing
REC	Research ethics committee
REM	Rapid eye movement (sleep)
RGF	Research governance framework
SCNMCR	Salford Centre for Nursing, Midwifery and Collaborative Research
SPEC	Student project ethics committee
SURGE	Service Users Research Group for England
TNF	Tumour necrosis factor
UAPMP	Unlinked anonymous prevalence monitoring programme
UKECA	United Kingdom Ethics Committee Authority
UREC	University research ethics committee
WMA	World Medical Association

Index

Page numbers in *italics* refer to figures and boxes.

Printed and bound by CPI Group (UK) Ltd, Croydon, CR0 4YY

03/10/2024

01040472-0002